YOUNG AGAIN!

GOD'S PLAN TO RESTORE YOUR SPIRIT OF YOUTH!

H. ALAN MUSHEGAN

Published by

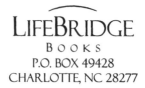

LIFEBRIDGE
B O O K S
P.O. BOX 49428
CHARLOTTE, NC 28277

Printed in the United States of America.

This book is dedicated to:

*– My father, Bishop Harry A. Mushegan,
and my mother, Myrtle Olene Mushegan,
who always believed.
– My sons, Alan, Aram and Ariel, who will
carry this message with power.
– My sisters Harolene and Janet, who with their
families have supported my dream.
– My church family, who believe in the vision.
– My departed friend, Charles Saia.
– Denise, who pressed me into "taking
it to the limit one more time."
– The Sweet Holy Spirit, whom
I cherish and serve.*

CONTENTS

INTRODUCTION

When I first read the Old Testament, I wondered, "How could great men and women of God still be energetic and vibrant at 120 years of age – and even older?"

If the Almighty could give strength and vitality to Moses, Joshua and David in the late years of their lives, what about you and me?

As I studied God's Word, He began to show me that age-reversal is not limited to the temporary treatment of medical doctors or psychologists, rather it is the divine will of the Almighty. From Genesis to Revelation we see how the Lord energizes His people – adding vigor and zest to their lives!

God doesn't simply give us a vision; He tells us to "*run* with it!"

Like an Eagle!

I'm excited you are reading this book. Why? Because I sincerely believe you are about to discover that the age on your birth certificate has absolutely no correlation to the life God wants you to experience.

It's true! The Lord desires for your youth be restored like the eagle's! This means you are going to soar above your problems and view life from a totally new perspective.

My friend, it's time to stop allowing Satan to dictate your health and happiness. As we will discover, the Lord was able to sustain the children of Israel in the wilderness without sickness and disease. Not only were their physical bodies renewed, the Bible says that even their clothing didn't wear out. It's no wonder they were able to throw a party in the desert!

The Most High God wants you to say goodbye to despondency and despair – and to experience dynamic living.

Let God Arise!

On these pages I want to share the connection between your faith and your youth. Hope, belief and expectation, instilled by God's Spirit, will result in uncommon strength and renewal.

I believe that as a result of this message, you will enter into a new relationship with the Lord – and feel God literally *arise* within you! There is absolutely nothing to compare with His power surging through your mind, heart and physical body.

You will also learn that in the Lord's divine plan, your setbacks are temporary. He wants you to see the big picture – clearing your thoughts of needless worry and your body of life-draining tension and stress.

We will answer these questions:

- How can I feed my faith instead of my fears?
- What is the secret of having "bulldog" tenacity?
- What are the requirements for becoming an overcomer?
- What is the divine relationship between total commitment and youthful living.
- What did Jesus say about becoming a child again?

In the final chapter I am going to pray with you for a brand new beginning. As a result, you can know what it is to start over – making this the first day of a marvelous new life.

Hang on! You are about to be *young again*!

Chapter 1

The Spirit of Youth

*C*an you imagine what it would be like to erase five, ten, twenty, or even *forty* years from your age? What you are about to discover is that in God's way of thinking, it is possible.

Since we are all guided by watches and clocks we constantly try to limit our activities – placing a time frame on what we can, should, and will do. Many shrug their shoulders, saying, "I've already lived most of my life and have probably accomplished all I'm going to achieve!"

The "spirit of youth" you will find on these pages has nothing to do with age. It is a *mind-set* and a *heart-set* – a spiritual renewal.

Instead of staying locked into a system dictated by

man, the Bible tells us: *"And be not conformed to this world: but be ye transformed by the renewing of your mind, that ye may prove what is that good, and acceptable, and perfect, will of God"* (Romans 12:2 KJV).

In other words, don't be bound by the way society operates or how modern culture thinks. Your life shouldn't be controlled by what Hollywood dictates or what MTV decides is "hip."

❖❖❖❖❖

YOUR LIFE SHOULDN'T BE CONTROLLED BY WHAT HOLLYWOOD DICTATES OR WHAT MTV DECIDES IS "HIP."

It's sad when trend-setters and marketing gurus determine what we wear, the kind of car we drive, even what we eat. Some people follow like sheep: "I saw it advertised on television so it must be good!"

Forever Young!

In the world's thought process, if you're 80 years old, you are living on borrowed time. Life is over!

Don't believe it. Forget about the date of birth on your driver's license. The only age that counts is the one the Almighty instills in your spirit and stamps on your heart. And, as you will learn, that age is forever young!

God's Word is referring to the spirit of youth when it says that instead of being *conformed* to this world, we are to be *transformed!* How? By the renewing of our mind.

When the touch of God comes upon you, there is *change!*

Let me put it bluntly: If you *conform* to the world's way of thinking, you'll become *deformed!* No longer will you be a person who is fresh, active and exciting.

In the process, the energy of your life will become diminished and you'll be *defused* – causing you to be *used* by everything and everyone around you.

Can you see the downward spiral in which Satan wants you trapped? Conformed – deformed – defused – then used!

This must not happen.

Dion Sanders, the former star of the Dallas Cowboys," was once asked, "What drove you to become such a great player in the NFL?"

CAN YOU SEE THE DOWNWARD SPIRAL IN WHICH SATAN WANTS YOU TRAPPED? CONFORMED – DEFORMED – DEFUSED – THEN USED!

He thought for a moment and answered, "When I was just a boy, I saw plenty of old men drinking beer on the corner. They'd say, 'If I had done this – or finished that – I could have really been somebody.'" Then he added, "I looked at their broken lives and told myself I wouldn't end up like that. I was determined to make it!"

Growing in the Desert

Why be defeated and give up on living? God can cause you to grow and prosper – anywhere, anytime and in any environment.

I love the words of the psalmist: *"The righteous will flourish like a palm tree, they will grow like a cedar of Lebanon"* (Psalm 92:12).

> **"THE RIGHTEOUS WILL FLOURISH LIKE A PALM TREE, THEY WILL GROW LIKE A CEDAR OF LEBANON."**
> - PSALM 93:12

Please understand, we are not righteous in and of ourselves. As an earthen vessel, I am certainly not what God expects me to be. In fact, without the Lord, I am a sinful, horrible person. But through Christ, I can put on *His* righteousness and experience not only *right* living, but *bright* living. With the Lord I have newness of life?

What does the Word say? I will "flourish like a palm tree!"

A palm can grow almost anywhere – even in an arid desert it survives. If you read the history of this amazing plant you'll find it can provide food, shelter and even clothing!

Your world may seem cracked and parched, and you worry, "Will anything meaningful ever happen to me?"

Hold on. God says you're going to flourish! When

everything seems impossible, new leaves and new life will begin to sprout. Even more, you will grow tall and sturdy – "like a cedar of Lebanon."

No "Lone Rangers!"

The next verse tells us what will happen when God renews our youthful spirit: Those who are *"planted in the house of the Lord...will flourish in the courts of our God"* (v.13).

I hope you realize that your Heavenly Father has placed you in the fellowship of believers for a purpose. He wants you to grow and mature in Him.

THERE ARE NO "LONE RANGERS" IN THE BODY OF CHRIST; WE ARE ALL CONNECTED AND JOINED TOGETHER.

There are no "Lone Rangers" in the body of Christ; we are all connected and joined together. I become concerned when a man or woman stands in a pulpit and announces, "Follow me. I'm the only one who is speaking the truth!"

No one is indispensable. We are linked together – not to defeat or destroy, but to edify, encourage, and lift each other up!

If you are a janitor or a secretary, understand God has placed you in that position and will give you the energy, inspiration and anointing to do what is necessary. The body of Christ requires doctors, lawyers, plumbers, electricians as well as pastors and evangelists. We are *all* in ministry!

The church God envisions is comprised of believers doing their assigned task with spirit and enthusiasm. It not only keeps them young, but causes the Great Commission to be aggressively fulfilled.

"Fat and Flourishing"

Remember, the Word tells us that if we are planted in the house of the Lord, we will blossom!

Look at what the psalmist said in the next verse:

"YOU MAY THINK I'M FADING AWAY, BUT I AM GOING TO GET FATTER!"

"They will still bear fruit in old age, they will stay fresh and green" (v.14). The King James Version says: *"... they shall be fat and flourishing."*

This means you're going to prosper. And it gives you the right to tell someone, "You may think I'm fading away, but I am going to get fatter!" Then you can explain God's "youth diet" to them!

The *fat* the Lord speaks of is the good of the land. It is what the Father gives you when you are linked and joined to what He wants to do in this generation.

16

"It's Coming!"

My friend, it doesn't matter whether a few gray hairs are starting to show, if wrinkles are lining your face, or you have pains in your back – when you accept God's spirit of youth, nothing can stop you.

When a pregnant woman goes through her gestation period of nine months, the father and the doctor can shake their heads in denial and say, "It not's coming!" but when the baby's time arrives – it's coming!

The same happens with you and me. When God places His spirit of youth within you and germinates a seed of hope and desire, get ready! It's going to produce at the appointed time, regardless of what others may say or do.

> ❖❖❖
>
> WHEN GOD PLACES HIS SPIRIT OF YOUTH WITHIN YOU AND GERMINATES A SEED OF HOPE AND DESIRE, GET READY!

What is the purpose in all of this? Keep reading. It is *"To show that the Lord is upright: he is my rock, and there is no unrighteousness in him"* (v.15 KJV).

When God makes a decision, it is always right! Some may criticize, "At your age, you don't deserve it. Your tired and worn out!"

They echoed those same words about Sarah, the elderly wife of Abraham. But when the Lord declares, "It will happen," that's all that counts. Even if your womb is dead, God will bring it back to life. He will recreate and restore what is needed for your future.

God's Renewal Process

Now is the time to come alive again! There's much more to life than waking up to an alarm clock, putting on your work clothes and facing another dreary day of drudgery.

THERE'S MUCH MORE TO LIFE THAN WAKING UP TO AN ALARM CLOCK, PUTTING ON YOUR WORK CLOTHES AND FACING ANOTHER DREARY DAY OF DRUDGERY.

God wants you to know this is a fresh new morning and you can accomplish something great in the Kingdom. That's what His renewal process is all about – so you will know *"his good, pleasing and perfect will"* (Romans 12:2).

There are far too many believers who call on the Name of Jesus, but never allow the Spirit of the Lord to revitalize their thinking so they can experience God's will for their lives.

No Fear!

You may ask, "How can I be young again? After all there is such a difference between the generations!"

Take a close look and you'll find the contrast is much

more than style and clothing. Young people confidently carry with them what we are discussing – the "spirit of youth." They have few worries and are basically optimistic about their future. In fact, one of the primary reasons young men and women enlist into the armed forces is because they are fearless – unafraid of dying. They feel invincible.

I remember the days when I played football and other contact sports. If I hit the ground, it was temporary. I bounced up and said, "Let's do it again!" Nothing was going to deter me!

I BOUNCED UP AND SAID, "LET'S DO IT AGAIN!" NOTHING WAS GOING TO DETER ME!

Tired? No Way!

As "young and foolish" teens, we would head to a beach in Florida with virtually no money. If anyone asked, "Where are you going to stay?" We would laugh and reply, "We'll find a place."

The word "tired" wasn't in my vocabulary. In those care-free days I would stay out practically all night and go to work at 7:00 A.M. the next morning. Whatever was happening, I wanted to be right in the middle of it.

Once, after working all day, my buddies and I went fishing on Lake Lanier, near Atlanta. In the middle of the night the engine on our boat conked out. Undaunted, we agreed, "Let's just have the current carry us so we can keep on fishing!" We didn't care.

It was still dark when we floated to shore – then walked for miles to find our car, making it back just in time for work the next morning.

Leaping Over Walls

What about today? Physically, my body has changed, but when I am inspired by a God-given idea, I am like an athlete on the starting blocks. My entire being springs to life in supernatural ways. When I am energized by God's Spirit, I feel like David, who exclaimed, *"For by thee I have run through a troop; and by my God have I leaped over a wall"* (Psalms 18:29 KJV).

I AM CONVINCED THAT WHEN GOD REJUVENATES YOUR "INNER MAN" EVERYTHING ABOUT YOU BECOMES NEW!

A good doctor can take care of your aging body, but what about your spirit? I am convinced that when God rejuvenates your "inner man" everything about you becomes new!

When you begin to move under God's anointing you will have the *spirit of youth*, regardless of your age! You will hear yourself saying, "I can do all things through Christ and Satan can't defeat me!"

The Giant's Challenge

If you truly desire something with all of your heart, absolutely nothing is going to stop you.

Let me take you back to one of the great confrontations in the Old Testament.

Picture the scene. On the side of one mountain, Saul, and the armies of Israel were gathered together. Across the valley, on another mountainside, were the Philistines – whose champion was Goliath.

The giant shouted across the valley, *"Why do you come out and line up for battle? Am I not a Philistine, and are you not the servants of Saul? Choose a man and have him come down to me. If he is able to fight and kill me, we will become your subjects; but if I overcome him and kill him, you will become our subjects and serve us"* (1 Samuel 17:8-9).

IF YOU TRULY DESIRE SOMETHING WITH ALL OF YOUR HEART, ABSOLUTELY NOTHING IS GOING TO STOP YOU.

King Saul's warriors were terrified. At the time, Jesse's youngest son, David, wasn't a soldier; he was tending sheep. When his father asked him to take some food to his older brothers in the encampment, David heard Goliath's challenge first-hand.

He also listened as the Israelites said: *"Do you see*

21

how this man keeps coming out? He comes out to defy Israel. The king will give great wealth to the man who kills him. He will also give him his daughter in marriage and will exempt his father's family from taxes in Israel" (v.25).

David asked the men standing near him, *"Who is this uncircumcised Philistine that he should defy the armies of the living God?"* (v.26).

"Who Do You Think You Are?"

Eliab, David's older brother, heard his words and was incensed. "What in the world are you doing here? Why aren't you tending your father's sheep?" he asked angrily. And he added: *"I know how conceited you are and how wicked your heart is; you came down only to watch the battle"* (v.28).

> "WHAT IN THE WORLD ARE YOU DOING HERE? WHY AREN'T YOU TENDING YOUR FATHER'S SHEEP?"

Even today, when you start to do something magnificent for the Lord, people will try to put you down before you start. They sneer, "Who do you think you are?"

David could have responded in kind, replying, "Just because you're older, and have on a suit of armor, you think you're a big shot!" but he didn't. Instead David simply replied, *"Now what have I done?...Can't I even speak?"* (v.29).

Those who heard David talking in such a manner, ran to tell King Saul – who immediately called for David.

"Only a Boy"

Suddenly, the spirit of youth rose up within David and he bravely said to Saul,

"Let no one lose heart on account of this Philistine; your servant will go and fight him" (v.32).

What was the king's response? Saul was shocked, and exclaimed, *"You are not able to go out against this Philistine and fight him; you are only a boy, and he has been a fighting man from his youth"* (v.33).

"YOU ARE NOT ABLE TO GO OUT AGAINST THIS PHILISTINE AND FIGHT HIM; YOU ARE ONLY A BOY, AND HE HAS BEEN A FIGHTING MAN FROM HIS YOUTH."
- 1 SAMUEL 17:33

David, trying to impress the king, bragged what a warrior he was as a shepherd. *"When a lion or a bear came and carried off a sheep from the flock, I went after it, struck it and rescued the sheep from its mouth. When it turned on me, I seized it by its hair, struck it and killed it"* (vv.34-35). Then he added, *"...this uncircumcised Philistine will be like one of them, because he has defied the armies of the living God"* (v.36).

David was convinced that the Lord who gave him strength to defeat the lion and bear would be with him in the face of Goliath. King Saul agreed, and told David, *"Go, and the Lord be with you"* (1 Samuel 17:37).

Five Smooth Stones

What an event it was! They tried to dress David with a full armor – helmet, breastplate and shield. But he protested. *"'I cannot go in these,' he said to Saul, 'because I am not used to them.' So he took them off"* (v.39).

❖•❖•❖•❖•

WITH NOTHING BUT A SLING IN HIS HAND, HE WALKED TOWARD THE GIANT.

Instead, David took five smooth stones from the brook and carefully placed them in his shepherd's bag. With nothing but a sling in his hand, he walked toward the giant.

Goliath couldn't believe his eyes. The Bible says, *"He looked David over and saw that he was only a boy, ruddy and handsome, and he despised him"* (v.42).

The Philistine wondered, "What is this? You send out a boy to do a man's job. Is there no man in Israel?" He taunted David: *"Am I a dog, that you come at me with sticks?"* (v.42).

Goliath cursed the young man, jeering, *"Come here...*

and I'll give your flesh to the birds of the air and the beasts of the field!" (v.44).

Oh, I love what David announced to the giant. He declared, *"You come against me with sword and spear and javelin, but I come against you in the name of the Lord Almighty, the God of the armies of Israel, whom you have defied"* (v.45).

What Goliath could not see was the Spirit of the Living God inside this young man.

✦•✦•✦•✦

WHAT GOLIATH COULD NOT SEE WAS THE SPIRIT OF THE LIVING GOD INSIDE THIS YOUNG MAN.

David believed in his heart, "With the Lord's help, I can defeat this enemy!"

Running Toward the Giant

For many days, thousands of men dressed in battle gear would not face this loud-mouth Philistine, yet here comes this young boy wearing a shepherd's garment who says, "Let me face this giant!"

You see, David wasn't weary. He had been alone with God, singing on the hillsides and in the pastures, rejoicing under the stars. Now, when Goliath spoke, he didn't hear the roar of a giant. He heard the still small voice of God in his heart reassuring him, "You can conquer this Philistine."

I can only imagine what this giant must have thought when he heard David boldly proclaim: *"This day the Lord will hand you over to me, and I'll strike you down and cut off your head. Today I will give the carcasses of the Philistine army to the birds of the air and the beasts of the earth, and the whole world will know that there is a God in Israel"* (v.46). He declared, *"for the battle is the Lord's, and he will give all of you into our hands"* (v.47).

WHEN YOU WALK IN THE SPIRIT OF YOUTH, THERE WILL ALWAYS BE THOSE WHO RIDICULE, NOT WANTING YOU TO TAKE AN ACTIVE ROLE IN ANYTHING.

After uttering those words, David literally *ran* toward the Philistine army to face Goliath. He had five stones, yet placed only one in his sling – and the giant was defeated!

Divine Encouragement

When you walk in the spirit of youth, there will always be those who ridicule, not wanting you to take an active role in anything. They would rather see you like themselves – dead to the world!

Ignore their criticism. Instead, take the advice of Paul the Apostle: *"Let no man despise thy youth; but be thou an example of the believers, in word, in conversation, in charity, in spirit, in faith, in purity"* (1 Timothy 4:12 KJV).

Today, God is still saying, "Do not let others condemn your *spirit* of youth!"

As you daily read the Word and receive the Lord's divine encouragement, step out of your comfort zone and begin to act on His promises.

•⋰•'⋰•'
TODAY, GOD IS STILL SAYING, "DO NOT LET OTHERS CONDEMN YOUR SPIRIT OF YOUTH!"

You may say, "I don't have anything to offer!" Well, David didn't either – there wasn't much ammunition in his shepherd's bag. But what a mighty victory!

It's Not Over!

My friend, I believe the Lord is preparing you to accomplish great feats in His Name.

It makes no difference whether Gabriel blows his horn today, next year or in the far distant future. The Lord tells us to work *"while it is day"* (John 9:4 KJV) because night is coming when no one can work.

Remember, *it's not over 'til it's over!*

In this time when evil and wickedness run rampant, God wants your spiritual zest and energy to be *"an example"* (1 Timothy 4:12). He desires that you demonstrate the joy and excitement of serving the Savior.

Regardless of your age, you can still show the world what it means to fight the good fight and overcome Satan. Forget what your physical body feels like, manifest a spirit that *demands* victory!

REGARDLESS OF YOUR AGE, YOU CAN STILL SHOW THE WORLD WHAT IT MEANS TO FIGHT THE GOOD FIGHT AND OVERCOME SATAN.

Tell the devil, "You may knock me down, but I'm not gonna stay down. With the Spirit's help, I am going to bounce back and keep fighting." As King Solomon wrote, *"For though a righteous man falls seven times, he rises again"* (Proverbs 24:16).

What Was it Like?

Just for a moment, reach back in your mind and try to remember what it felt like:

- When you scored the goal that gave your team a victory.
- When you turned the key on the ignition of your first car.
- When you truly fell in love.
- When you gave your heart to the Lord.

Don't just recall those moments as ancient history;

start to re-live them again. Once more, grasp the emotions and walk in that same joy and excitement.

You may say, "But I have changed. I am getting older."

That is not a valid excuse. God declares, *"For I am the Lord, I change not"* (Malachi 3:6 KJV). If you are His child, you already have eternity in your heart and you won't change either!

Living Water

What makes it possible for you to become young again? It's the renewing spirit of the Holy Ghost – the *paraclete* (or Comforter) promised by Christ before He returned to heaven. It is His breath flowing through us that gives us new life.

WHAT MAKES IT POSSIBLE FOR YOU TO BECOME YOUNG AGAIN? IT'S THE RENEWING SPIRIT OF THE HOLY GHOST.

Far too many believers are sitting around aimlessly, waiting for God to take them home, when they need to be drinking of the Living Water, and eating of the Bread of Life.

The spirit of youth says, "I want it *now!*" Instead of simply talking about what *might* be possible, realize that God has already given you the power and authority to take dominion. He wants you to speak these things into existence and possess the land!

No-Limit Living

More than once I've heard people with "underprivileged" backgrounds complain, "But you don't understand; I haven't had the same opportunities as others. I have limitations!"

♦•¦•♦

WHEN GOD INFUSES YOU WITH HIS SPIRIT OF YOUTH, YOU CAN CONQUER ALL THINGS.

Friend, it makes no difference where you were born, your educational experience or economic status. When God infuses you with His Spirit of youth, you can conquer all things. Listen to what Jesus declares: *"Everything is possible for him who believes"* (Mark 9:23).

If young people believe they can climb the highest mountains, why can't you? The Lord is saying, "Believe it and receive it." He wants you to draw a line in the sand and stand your ground. Claim what is rightfully yours!

Again, the Lord says: *"With man this is impossible, but not with God; all things are possible with God"* (Mark 10:27).

"Yea and Amen!"

How do you see the Almighty? Do you perceive God as omnipotent, all powerful? Or do you view Him with barriers and limitations?

For me, when the Lord gives a decree it is already accomplished; it is "yea and amen!"

If God says He is going to open the door to a new job, start writing your resume. If He tells you that you're going to find a wonderful Christian husband, start picking out your wedding dress! Rest assured that what He says will come to pass.

You may be sick in body, yet if the Lord declares you're going to live, the devil has no say in the matter.

When God whispers "You're going to make it!" you can smile at your unbelieving friends. You *will* triumph!

With the Spirit of the Father, you are young again! Everything is possible!

CHAPTER 2

KEEP ON PARTYING!

Wow! An 80-year-old man leading a celebration in the middle of a desert? That's what Moses did after he escaped from Pharoah and led the children of Israel out of the bondage of Egypt.

If Moses were living today, someone would probably grab him by the beard and say, "Look, mister, you're far too old to be taking three million people on a trek through the wilderness. Have you lost your mind?"

After all, Moses was no spring chicken! At the age of 40 he left Egypt and spent the next four decades tending sheep on the backside of the mountain. God was preparing him for perhaps the greatest adventure in recorded history.

Now, at 80, he stood before Pharoah, demanding "Let my people go!"

A "Burning" Encounter

How could Moses speak with such authority? Many years earlier, this old man had an encounter with God that transformed his life. While he was tending the flock of his father-in-law, Jethro, the angel of the Lord appeared to him in flames of fire from within a bush.

GOD CALLED HIM FROM WITHIN THE BUSH: "MOSES! MOSES!" HE REPLIED, "HERE I AM!"

Moses saw that even though the bush was ablaze, it didn't burn up. When he moved closer to observe, God called him from within the bush: "Moses! Moses!"

He replied, "Here I am!"

Then the Lord cautioned, *"Do not come any closer ...Take off your sandals, for the place where you are standing is holy ground"* (Exodus 3:5).

He was in the presence of the Almighty!

"I AM!"

God also told Moses he had heard the cry of the Israelites and *"I am sending you to Pharaoh to bring my people the Israelites out of Egypt"* (v.10).

What an awesome order! However, Moses had more immediate things to worry about. At the time, he wasn't even the leader of his own people.

Moses said to the Lord, *"Suppose I go to the Israel- ites and say to them, 'The God of your fathers has sent me to you,' and they ask me, 'What is his name?' Then what shall I tell them?"* (v.13).

God replied to Moses, *"I AM WHO I AM. This is what you are to say to the Israel- ites: 'I AM has sent me to you'"* (v.14).

The Lord was saying to the future leader of Israel, "Everything you can think of, and everything you need, I AM!"

THE LORD WAS SAYING TO THE FUTURE LEADER OF ISRAEL, "EVERYTHING YOU CAN THINK OF, AND EVERYTHING YOU NEED, I AM!"

- "If you need a warrior, I AM!"
- "If you need a healer, I AM!"
- "If you need a deliverer, I AM!"

Walking in that authority, the Israelites accepted Moses as God's appointed leader and miracles began to occur. Great plagues fell upon the people of Egypt until a frustrated Pharoah finally summoned Moses and said, *"Up! Leave my people, you and the Israelites! Go, worship the Lord as you have requested. Take your flocks and herds, as you have said, and go"* (Exodus 12:31-32).

Pharoah had seen enough and wanted these people gone!

Crisis at the Red Sea

On their journey, the Lord guided the children of Israel with a cloud by day and a pillar of fire by night. However, by the time they reached the Red Sea, Pharoah realized he had made a horrendous mistake. He exclaimed, *"What have we done? We have let the Israelites go and lost their services!"* (Exodus 14:6).

After all, cheap labor was hard to find!

Pharoah quickly summoned his entire army together and they set out to recapture the Israelites. And when the children of Israel looked over their shoulders and saw the chariots, horsemen and troops of the Egyptians, they were terrified.

WHEN THE CHILDREN OF ISRAEL LOOKED OVER THEIR SHOULDERS AND SAW THE CHARIOTS, HORSEMEN AND TROOPS OF THE EGYPTIANS, THEY WERE TERRIFIED.

They cried out to Moses: *"What have you done to us by bringing us out of Egypt?...It would have been better for us to serve the Egyptians than to die in the desert!"* (vv.11-12).

36

The Waters Parted!

At the edge of the water – and on the verge of extinction – Moses answered the people: *"Do not be afraid. Stand firm and you will see the deliverance the Lord will bring you today. The Egyptians you see today you will never see again. The Lord will fight for you; you need only to be still"* (vv.13-14).

At that moment God told Moses to raise his staff and stretch his hand over the sea. When he did, the Lord began to push back the water with such a strong wind it divided the sea and the Israelites crossed on dry ground. The Bible records there was *"a wall of water on their right and on their left"* (v.22).

> "DO NOT BE AFRAID. STAND FIRM AND YOU WILL SEE THE DELIVERANCE THE LORD WILL BRING YOU TODAY."
> - EXODUS 14:13

The Egyptians, of course, were in hot pursuit. And before long all of Pharaoh's army followed them into the sea.

On the other side, God told Moses: *"Stretch out your hand over the sea so that the waters may flow back over the Egyptians and their chariots and horsemen"* (v.26).

Suddenly, Pharoah's entire army drowned. *"Not one of them survived"* (v.28).

37

Time to Celebrate!

The people saw the power of God in action, and as a result, they put their trust in the Lord – and in His servant, Moses.

I'M SURE THEY DIDN'T NEED AN EXCUSE, BUT THE BIBLE RECORDS THEY HAD A PARTY! THEY CELEBRATED!

I'm sure they didn't need an excuse, but the Bible records they had a party! They celebrated!

Moses, and the children of Israel, gathered together and began to sing. What a glorious sound of victory it must have been as they lifted their voices to Jehovah.

Listen to their words:

"I will sing to the Lord, for he is highly exalted.
The horse and its rider he has hurled into the sea.
The Lord is my strength and my song;
he has become my salvation.
He is my God, and I will praise him,
my father's God, and I will exalt him.
The Lord is a warrior; the Lord is his name.
Pharaoh's chariots and his army
he has hurled into the sea.
The best of Pharaoh's officers are
drowned in the Red Sea.

The deep waters have covered them;
they sank to the depths like a stone.
Your right hand,
O Lord, was majestic in power"
(Exodus 15:1-6).

It wasn't just the men who were jubilant. The Bible says that Miriam the prophetess, Aaron's sister, took a tambourine in her hand, *"and all the women followed her, with tambourines and dancing. Miriam sang to them: 'Sing to the Lord, for he is highly exalted. The horse and its rider he has hurled into the sea'"* (Exodus 15:20-21).

What a party!

Uncommon Strength

For the next 40 years, Moses followed the Lord's command and led the people. Finally, on mount Nebo, his days came to an end. Here's what is so amazing: during the grueling ordeal this great man of God never lost his youth! Even surrounded by doubting, rebellious people, he still maintained his vitality.

EVEN SURROUNDED BY DOUBTING, REBELLIOUS PEOPLE, HE STILL MAINTAINED HIS VITALITY.

The Word records, *"Moses was a hundred and twenty*

years old when he died, yet his eyes were not weak nor his strength gone" (Deuteronomy 34:7). The King James Version says, *"his eye was not dim, nor his natural force abated."*

In other words, Moses functioned like a man half his age – or even younger.

You may say, "Well, people lived much longer in those days." That's not true – only *some* enjoyed a long life span, and only because God lengthened their days. Many died early because of disease and lack of medical care.

❖❖❖

MOSES FUNCTIONED LIKE A MAN HALF HIS AGE - OR EVEN YOUNGER.

Do you believe the Lord loves you as much as He loved Moses? Can He do the same for you? Since *"God is no respecter of persons"* (Acts 10:34 KJV), of course He can!

You Won't Wear Out!

Let me share one of the most overlooked facts that took place in the wilderness. Toward the end of their journey, Moses reminded the people how they were fed with manna from heaven, and *"Your clothes did not wear out and your feet did not swell during these forty years"* (Deuteronomy 8:4).

What a miracle! The people were walking in the hot

desert sand, yet their feet didn't feel the effects of the constant travel.

Can you imagine buying a dress, a suit and a pair of shoes and keeping them for 40 years? Nothing wore out!

I hope you realize that if the Lord can keep man-made garments fresh and new, He can do even more with your physical body. According to the Word, if you are part of God's plan, you won't wear out! "Your "natural forces" will not abate.

Why give up before the celebration even begins?

Perceive It!

Moses walked in the energy of God's power because the Lord revealed a clear purpose for his life. In other words, he perceived what God expected and lived accordingly.

You already possess the potential for greatness, yet if you see yourself as a failure, that's exactly the way you'll be received.

> MOSES WALKED IN THE ENERGY OF GOD'S POWER BECAUSE THE LORD REVEALED A CLEAR PURPOSE FOR HIS LIFE.

Jesus and His disciples were traveling to the villages near Caesarea Philippi. On the way He asked them, *"Who do people say I am?"* (Mark 8:27). The Lord wanted to know, "Who do they perceive me to be?"

The Son of God knew that if the people accepted Him as the Christ, then He would be the Messiah to them.

The Restorer of Youth

Your mind is a powerful instrument. When pharmaceutical companies test new drugs they enroll people in a research program and give half of those with the targeted ailment a placebo – a "sugar pill." It's amazing, but many times those who take the placebo start improving.

When your world seems to be crashing down upon you, start "seeing" the Lord lifting you up, sustaining you. Believe the words of the psalmist are written for you: *"A thousand shall fall at thy side, and ten thousand at thy right hand; but it shall not come nigh thee"* (Psalm 91:7).

ISN'T IT TIME WE VIEW THE LORD TO BE THE TRUE GIVER OF LIFE, THE MASTER OF ALL THINGS, THE RESTORER OF YOUTH?

Why is this possible? Because you perceive Him to be God!

Isn't it time we view the Lord to be the true Giver of Life, the Master of All Things, the Restorer of Youth?

The Father not only plans for you to celebrate, He

will give you the vigor and vitality to make it through the midnight hour. He has seen your days of doubt and depression, and now your hour has come.

This is not the time to be timid or afraid: *"For God hath not given us the spirit of fear; but of power, and of love, and of a sound mind"* (2 Timothy 1:7).

He wants you to rejoice!

David's Party

When the Lord does something special in your life, it's time for a jubilee!

David did just that when he was named King of Israel and the Ark of God was once again restored. Here's how the Bible describes the party that followed: *"David and the whole house of Israel were celebrating with all their might before the Lord, with songs and with harps, lyres, tambourines...and cymbals"* (2 Samuel 6:5).

WHEN THE LORD DOES SOMETHING SPECIAL IN YOUR LIFE, IT'S TIME FOR A JUBILEE!

In the next generation, after Solomon dedicated the great temple, all of Israel celebrated *"for seven days and seven days more, fourteen days in all"* (1 Kings 8:65). The people were, *"joyful and glad in heart for all the good things the Lord had done"* (v.66).

Joy in Heaven

The rejoicing we read about in the Old Testament can't compare with what happens when you ask Christ to be your Lord and Savior. At that precise moment, a tremendous celebration takes place in heaven.

THE REJOICING WE READ ABOUT IN THE OLD TESTAMENT CAN'T COMPARE WITH WHAT HAPPENS WHEN YOU ASK CHRIST TO BE YOUR LORD AND SAVIOR.

Jesus describes what occurs by telling this story. He said, *"Suppose one of you has a hundred sheep and loses one of them. Does he not leave the ninety-nine in the open country and go after the lost sheep until he finds it? And when he finds it, he joyfully puts it on his shoulders and goes home. Then he calls his friends and neighbors together and says, 'Rejoice with me; I have found my lost sheep.' I tell you that in the same way there will be more rejoicing in heaven over one sinner who repents than over ninety-nine righteous persons who do not need to repent"* (Luke 15:4-7).

Then He added one more example: *"Suppose a woman has ten silver coins and loses one. Does she not light a lamp, sweep the house and search carefully until she finds it? And when she finds it, she calls her friends and neighbors together and says, 'Rejoice with me; I have found my lost coin.' In the same way, I tell you, there is rejoicing in the presence of the angels of God over one sinner who repents"* (Luke 15:8-10).

"Let's Have a Feast!"

Your decision to repent and turn your life over to the Lord is a signal for the angels to start singing. Even on earth, it's a time to rejoice. When the prodigal son returned home, his father, said, *"Quick! Bring the best robe and put it on him. Put a ring on his finger and sandals on his feet. Bring the fattened calf and kill it. Let's have a feast and celebrate. For this son of mine was dead and is alive again; he was lost and is found"* (Luke 15:22-24).

YOUR DECISION TO REPENT AND TURN YOUR LIFE OVER TO THE LORD IS A SIGNAL FOR THE ANGELS TO START SINGING.

What a time of joy and delight that was!

The Great Wedding Party!

I hope you realize that at this very moment, your Father is preparing a festive event beyond anything you can imagine. It's going to be the wedding party of all time!

John's revelation of heaven gives us a preview. He writes: *"Let us rejoice and be glad and give him glory! For the wedding of the Lamb has come, and his bride has made herself ready. Fine linen, bright and clean, was given her to wear"* (Revelation 19:7-8).

As a believer, you have been presented with a special invitation: *"Blessed are those who are invited to the wedding supper of the Lamb!"* (Revelation 19:9).

The Lord doesn't need an exhausted, tired, complaining bride, rather one who is excited about an eternal future with Him.

Get ready for a divine party that will never end!

CHAPTER 3

STILL CRAZY
AFTER ALL
THESE YEARS!

If you are a Bible-believing, God-fearing, born-again Christian, don't be surprised when people think you've lost your marbles!

Those you work with may look with disapproval when you take a moment to bow your head in prayer before lunch. Even some of your relatives may wonder why you attend church so often – and constantly talk about what Jesus is doing in your life.

When people think you are a weirdo, take a deep breath, smile, and say with the Apostle Paul, *"We are fools for Christ"* (1 Corinthians 4:10). You see, *"God chose the foolish things of the world to shame the wise; God chose the weak things of the world to shame the strong"* (1 Corinthians 1:27).

If people want to say I have lost my senses by serving Christ, I'll wear it as a badge of honor. In the words of Paul Simon's hit song, I'm *"Still Crazy After All These Years!"*

"Hold On!"

More than once, the children of Israel thought Moses was out of his mind, leading them on a wild goose chase through the sweltering heat and sizzling sand. They complained, *"We remember the fish we ate in Egypt at no cost – also the cucumbers, melons, leeks, onions and garlic. But now we have lost our appetite; we never see anything but this manna!"* (Numbers 11:5-6).

"HOLD ON!" MOSES WOULD ENCOURAGE, "WE ARE ALMOST THERE!"

"Hold on!" Moses would encourage, "We are almost there!"

After four long decades in the wilderness, Moses and the disgruntled people he led were getting close to the Promised Land. There numbers hadn't dwindled. Scripture records they still had *"six hundred thousand men on foot"* (Numbers 11:21) – and counting the women and children, the number exceeded three million.

"Milk and Honey"

The Lord asked Moses to send twelve spies (one man from each tribe) to secretly explore the land of Canaan and bring back a report. Moses wanted them to *"See what the land is like and whether the people who live there are strong or weak, few or many. What kind of land do they live in? Is it good or bad? What kind of towns do they live in? Are they unwalled or fortified? How is the soil? Is it fertile or poor? Are there trees on it or not? Do your best to bring back some of the fruit of the land. (It was the season for the first ripe grapes.)"* (Numbers 13:18-20).

Forty days later the spies returned and presented their report to the entire Israelite community who had gathered on the Desert of Paran. They brought with them samples of the bountiful fruit of the land – huge grapes and delicious pomegranates. And they told of a land flowing with *"milk and honey"* (v.27).

THEY BROUGHT WITH THEM SAMPLES OF THE BOUNTIFUL FRUIT OF THE LAND - HUGE GRAPES AND DELICIOUS POMEGRANATES.

Then came the negative news: *"But the people who live there are powerful, and the cities are fortified and very large. We even saw descendants of Anak there"* (v.28). These were gigantic people.

Was he Crazy?

Of the twelve spies, only two – Joshua and Caleb – had an optimistic view of the situation. Immediately, Caleb stood up and silenced the frightened throng, declaring, *"We should go up and take possession of the land, for we can certainly do it"* (v.30).

They thought he was crazy!

The others on the expedition publicly exclaimed, *"We can't attack those people; they are stronger than we are"* (v.31). And, *"The land we explored devours those living in it. All the people we saw there are of great size...We seemed like grasshoppers in our own eyes, and we looked the same to them"* (vv.32-33).

I CAN HEAR THEM CRYING, "WE'RE GRASSHOPPERS! THEY'RE GOING TO EAT US UP!"

The bad report spread through the Israelites like a virus. That night all the people of the community *"raised their voices and wept aloud"* (Numbers 14:1).

I can hear them crying, "We're grasshoppers! They're going to eat us up!"

Two Exceptions

Why were they weeping? These ten spies, and the people who believed them, dwelled on their weakness instead of their strength. They focused on their inabilities instead of their abilities – looking at their flesh instead of their faith.

As we will discover, because they had no vision, they received no possession.

God was so displeased at the unbelieving children of Israel, He declared *"...not one of the men who saw my glory and the miraculous signs I performed in Egypt and in the desert but who disobeyed me and tested me ten times – not one of them will ever see the land I promised on oath to their forefathers. No one who has treated me with contempt will ever see it"* (vv.22-23).

There were two exceptions – Joshua and Caleb. The Lord said, *"But because my servant Caleb has a different spirit and follows me wholeheartedly, I will bring him into the land he went to, and his descendants will inherit it"* (v.24). And He declared the same about Joshua (v.30).

WHAT GOD SAW IN THESE TWO MEN WAS AN "I CAN DO IT!" DETERMINATION - A "NOTHING CAN STOP ME!" ATTITUDE.

They Believed!

What God saw in these two men was an "I can do it!" determination – a "Nothing can stop me!" attitude. It was the spirit of youth! Scripture records that the Lord told

Moses to lay his hand on Joshua – *"a man in whom is the spirit"* (Numbers 27:18).

Please understand that Joshua and Caleb were among the millions who had seen the cloud by day and fire by night – and who had witnessed the parting of the Red Sea. Like everyone else, they had been miraculously fed by manna and drank water that sprang out of a rock.

What made the difference between these two men and the others? They *believed!*

Inch by Inch!

The Promised Land wasn't handed to Joshua and Caleb on a silver platter. They had to fight for every inch of it – and it took another 45 years. There were battles at Jericho and Ai, and conflicts with the Gibeonites, the Amorites and so many more. Read Chapter 12 of Joshua and you'll find the names of 31 kings who were defeated.

THE PROMISED LAND WASN'T HANDED TO JOSHUA AND CALEB ON A SILVER PLATTER. THEY HAD TO FIGHT FOR EVERY INCH OF IT - AND IT TOOK ANOTHER 45 YEARS.

Joshua stayed true to the vision and kept moving forward! When he was well advanced in years, the Lord said to him, *"You are very old, and there are still very large areas of land to be taken over"* (Joshua 13:1). The same God who gave him the promise, showered him with strength and energy for the task ahead.

Finally, after the conflicts were almost over and the land was ready to be totally possessed, Caleb reminisced with Joshua about the time Moses sent them to explore Canna. He recalled, *"I was forty years old when Moses the servant of the Lord sent*

THE SAME GOD WHO GAVE HIM THE PROMISE, SHOWERED HIM WITH STRENGTH AND ENERGY FOR THE TASK AHEAD.

me...to explore the land. And I brought him back a report according to my convictions, but my brothers who went up with me made the hearts of the people melt with fear. I, however, followed the Lord my God wholeheartedly" (Joshua 14:8).

Still Going Strong!

Caleb remembered Moses telling him that the land on which his feet had walked *"will be your inheritance and that of your children forever"* (v.9) because he had followed the Lord.

Then Caleb observed, *"...just as the Lord promised, he has kept me alive for forty-five years since the time he said this to Moses, while Israel moved about in the desert. So here I am today, eighty-five years old!"* (v.10).

Now he was ready! The wicked generations – those who thought he was crazy – had died off and Caleb felt young again! He declared, *"I am still as strong today as the day Moses sent me out; I'm just as vigorous to go out to battle now as I was then"* (v.11).

"I'm Not a Grasshopper!

This anointed man followed a timeless, limitless God. Caleb – whose name in Hebrew means *forcible* – had a faith much greater than his age. He not only had God's strength, but also His promise. That's why he could look at the land of Hebron and declare: *"Now therefore give me this mountain, whereof the Lord spake in that day"* (v.12 KJV).

AT THE AGE OF 85, CALEB WASN'T READY TO DRINK WARM MILK, WRAP UP IN A BLANKET, AND DIE.

We need to understand the mountain presented problems – it was a land with fortified cities ruled by the Anakites. Yet the Lord blessed Caleb and gave him the land as an inheritance *"because he followed the Lord, The God of Israel, wholeheartedly"* (v.14).

At the age of 85, Caleb wasn't ready to drink warm milk, wrap up in a blanket, and die. Others saw defeat, yet he was ready for battle. He said, "I am not a grasshopper. I'm a mountain taker!"

Every Promise Fulfilled

What happened to Joshua? Under his leadership, *"the Lord gave Israel all the land he had sworn to give their forefathers, and they took possession of it and settled there...Not one of all the Lord's good promises to the house of Israel failed; every one was fulfilled"* (Joshua 21:43,45).

Until he drew his final breath, Joshua was an energetic leader. Scripture records that he *"died at the age of a hundred and ten. And they buried him in the land of his inheritance"* (Joshua 24:29-30).

What a glorious life he led!

"It's Mine!"

When God gives you a vision, forget the nay-sayers and critics. Prepare for battle and start marching ahead. It is the only way you'll receive your promise.

Joshua and Caleb had to move past doubt and disbelief – even the giants. As Caleb exclaimed, "That's my mountain and nothing's going to stop me – not my adversaries nor my age!"

You too must stand up to Satan and say: "No weapon

> WHEN GOD GIVES YOU A VISION, FORGET THE NAY-SAYERS AND CRITICS.

formed against me shall prosper! What God declared He will deliver! It's mine!"

Be Careful?

There will always be people who question, "What is this business of 'walking by faith?' Why don't you think rationally?"

My friend, you can never try to outguess the ways of an unseen God?

THE LORD IS LOOKING FOR RISK-TAKING, FAITH-WALKING, MOUNTAIN-CLIMBING BELIEVERS.

When they tell you, "Just be careful," remember the Word tells us, *"Be careful for nothing; but in every thing by prayer and supplication with thanksgiving let your requests be made known unto God"* (Philippians 4:6).

Forget about those who try to burst your balloon, asking, "What's the use? You'd better stop trying!"

If you listen to their misguided advice you will never walk in God's fullness and receive the inheritance He has promised.

What Will He Say?

The Lord is looking for risk-taking, faith-walking, mountain-climbing believers. Regardless of what people may think about you here on earth, there's only one opinion that truly matters. What will the Lord declare when you stand before Him on that Great Day?

As a servant of the Most High, you will hear Him say – as He surely announced to Joshua and Caleb – "Well done, thou good and faithful servant. Come into the Kingdom and rest!"

For eternity you will exclaim, "I'm still praising after all these years!"

CHAPTER 4

RUNNING
WITH HORSES!

In Benin City, Nigeria, a tiny baby was born to impoverished parents. His name was Benson. The sickly infant, born with a deformity, was always fainting.

Tragically, when the child was only 18 months old – as a result of his constant illness – his father ordered the mother to throw him on a garbage heap where he was left to die.

Somehow, this rejected boy survived and eventually became a servant on a farm – where he was denied a formal education. In his teens, while playing soccer with his friends, a local preacher stopped by to tell them the story of Jesus, and Benson's life was totally transformed.

The young man became a zealous soul-winner, and one night he had a vison from the Lord. God told him "I have called you to take My message around the world. Preach the Gospel and I will confirm My Word with signs following."

"What's the Secret?"

The world came to know this man as Archbishop Benson Idahosa, a spiritual giant who established over 6,000 churches in Africa – many with several thousand members. God used him to shake nations for Christ.

"I CAN'T UNDERSTAND YOU AMERICANS. YOU HAVE EVERYTHING AND DO NOTHING WITH IT!"

Before the Lord called him home in 1998, I had the opportunity to spend some time with this inspiring man. I asked him, "How were you able to go from your humble beginnings and build a church seating 10,000 in your home town? What's the secret?"

His answer was simple, yet profound. Benson replied, "I kept reaching *up!*" Then he added, "I can't understand you Americans. You have everything and do nothing with it!"

He couldn't comprehend our mentality of spiritual complacency – and truly believed we should aggressively conquer all things through Christ – regardless of the obstacles Satan throws in our way.

The Vultures

Once, when Idahosa was holding a crusade, the village witch doctors began to curse the people who attended the meetings and vowed to shut him down. You may not think these evil men possess any power, but strange things happen when people link up with the devil.

Several thousand were attending the crusade when the witch doctors commanded vultures to come and attack the people. As Benson described it, "These creatures came diving out of the sky and literally attacked many in the audience, hurting them. The people began to scatter."

Benson grabbed the microphone and announced, "I want everyone to be back here tomorrow night." Then he added, "In the Name of Jesus, if one vulture comes to the meeting, you witch doctors will die! Did you hear me? You will *die!*"

"IN THE NAME OF JESUS, IF ONE VULTURE COMES TO THE MEETING, YOU WITCH DOCTORS WILL DIE!"

The next evening, only one vulture was visible – and it was perched on the branch of a tree far away from the crowd. But the best part of the story is that many of those same witch doctors came to the altar and gave their hearts to Christ. They realized there was almighty power in God's Son, Jesus.

Benson Idahosa, may have been discarded on a garbage heap, but he didn't remain there. This deformed weakling, grew to be strong because he found Someone greater than himself.

"Run With Achievers!"

I will never forget the advice he gave me: "Alan," he said, "if you want to be successful, never hang around with unsuccessful people. You've got to take God as your partner and run with achievers!"

IF YOU'RE EXHAUSTED FROM RUNNING WITH AVERAGE PEOPLE, HOW IN THE WORLD ARE YOU GOING TO KEEP UP WHEN THE BATTLE GET'S ROUGH?

That word was not only practical, it was spiritual. The Bible tells us we need to be *running with horses!*

The prophet Jeremiah asks this question: *"If you have raced with men on foot and they have worn you out, how can you compete with horses? If you stumble in safe country, how will you manage in the thickets by the Jordan?"* (Jeremiah 12:5).

If you're exhausted from running with average people, how in the world are you going to keep up when the battle gets rough? You'd better be in shape for the race ahead.

Choose your company carefully. You can't run with the horses if you are hanging around with mules!

Train for the Battle

I believe we have languished so long in the land of plenty that we've become spiritually "soft." When it comes to fulfilling the Great Commission, we say, "Let the pastors and evangelists do it. After all, that's what we pay them for!"

Oh, how I wish every believer could, just for a moment, be transported to a land where religious persecution exists – to experience first-hand what it is like to be ridiculed and even put in prison for speaking the name of Jesus.

IT'S TIME TO START TRAINING OUR MIND, HEART, SOUL AND BODY TO BE IN PEAK CONDITION FOR THE BATTLE AHEAD.

If this easy life wearies us, how are we going to respond when trouble comes? It's time to start training our mind, heart, soul and body to be in peak condition for the battle ahead.

Perhaps you need to ask the Lord to give you a "kick start" that will force you from your bed of complacency. There's so much more you can accomplish – and God will give you the zest and zeal to do it!

Run With the Vision

Personally, I've made my decision to walk in the power and promises of the Father. With child-like faith and expectation, I believe if God says it, I can obtain it!

What about you? Have you made that same declaration? You may still be saying, "Alan, it's not that easy. You don't know what my life has been like!"

Is it worse than being discarded on a trash pile? Is it more tragic than being a slave?

DON'T JUST RECEIVE THE VISION - RUN WITH IT!

Your future is not what you say, rather what God declares – and according to the Word, you have a great potential. You may ask, "What am I supposed to be doing with my life?"

Now is the time to fall on your face before the Lord and stay in His presence until He begins to reveal a clear picture of your future – yes, a vision of His plan and purpose for you.

Then, when the curtain has been rolled back and you "see" what the Lord expects, do what the Word says: *"Write the vision, and make it plain upon tables, that he may run that readeth it"* (Habakkuk 2:2 KJV).

What a statement! Don't just receive the vision – *run* with it! Get moving until His blueprint for your future is turned into something tangible!

Total Trust

Before you can run with the horses, you've got to visualize yourself moving ahead – invigorated by His power.

Where does it begin? With faith and trust! Scripture declares, *"And without faith it is impossible to please God, because anyone who comes to him must believe that he exists and that he rewards those who earnestly seek him"* (Hebrews 11:6).

THE LORD EXPECTS YOUR UNSWERVING CONFIDENCE, YOUR TOTAL TRUST.

The Lord expects your *unswerving* confidence, your total trust. Embracing His belief system is the only way to run the race ahead.

Not only do I believe the Creator rules the affairs of man, but according to His Word, if I diligently seek Him, that same God is going to reward, bless and heal me, and cause me to prosper.

Make it Personal

Just think how much farther and faster you can progress when the Lord's mighty hand is holding yours – leading and guiding you forward.

Many believe God can perform miracles for others, but aren't sure He can do it for them. They pray for the healing of someone they love, yet question if He will touch their own body.

There comes a time when you must look up to heaven and say, "God, Your Word declares You are a rewarder of those who earnestly seek You – and I am seeking You with all of my heart and soul."

When that prayer rises from the depths of your spirit, the Lord will not only hear you, He will begin to bless you – *abundantly!*

Add Faith

The same God who brought the children of Israel out of the land of Egypt with signs, with wonders and *"a strong hand"* (Jeremiah 32:21), will quicken your body.

Start believing in God's strength – for you! Or, to say it another way, *strengthen your belief so that God's hand will work!* It is your faith that moves the heart of the Almighty.

IT IS YOUR FAITH THAT MOVES THE HEART OF THE ALMIGHTY.

In medical science, when you mix certain ingredients together it creates a product that can result in great benefits. When you read God's Word, you will discover the required components – and one of them is faith. It is part of the belief structure that allows the Father to work on your behalf.

The Power of Belief

Without faith, everything slows to a grinding halt. From the moment Jesus began His public ministry there were mighty miracles:

- He delivered a demon-possessed man in the synagogue at Capernaum (Mark 1:21-26).
- Simon's mother-in-law was healed of a fever (vv.29-31).
- He said "Be clean" to a leper and he was completely healed (vv.40-41).
- To the paralytic, He declared, "Take up your bed and walk" – and the man walked! (Mark 2:1-12).
- On the shores of the Sea of Galilee, He brought a dead girl back to life (Mark 5:35-42).

Yet look at what occurred when Jesus returned to His hometown – Nazareth. Instead of acceptance there was doubt. Accompanied by His disciples, He began to teach on the Sabbath in the synagogue and the people began to question.

"'Where did this man get these things?' they asked. 'What's this wisdom that has been given him, that he even does miracles! Isn't this the carpenter? Isn't this Mary's son and the brother of James, Joseph, Judas and

Simon?...And they took offense at him" (Mark 6:2-3).

What was the result of their unbelief? Scripture records: *"He could not do any miracles there, except lay his hands on a few sick people and heal them, and he was amazed at their lack of faith"* (vv.5-6).

You see, the Lord requires an atmosphere of belief.

Starve Your Doubts!

Beginning right now, start feeding your faith instead of your fears.

If you want to get rid of your anxieties and worries, don't entertain them. It's like giving food to a stray cat – once you do, that little animal is going to keep showing up at your house. The same thing happens when you feed your fears – they don't go away. Exhausted, you put your head on your pillow at night and all of a sudden here they come again! Your mind is overcome with doubt, worry and anxiety.

BEGINNING RIGHT NOW, START FEEDING YOUR FAITH INSTEAD OF YOUR FEARS.

Fear shows up because you fed it.

Remember this: If there is something you don't understand, turn it over to the Lord. The reason you can trust God with your fears is because He knows all about them. Say to the Lord: "I may not understand, but You do. I know You are going to help me walk through the valley of the shadow of death. The path is dark, but Lord, You give me light!"

"Trust Me!"

If you have ever raised a teenager you no doubt have heard them say, "But why can't I go to the party?" Or, "Why won't you let me go to the movies with Billy?"

When you reply with an emphatic "No," the usual response is, "I don't understand!"

As a parent, you answer, "Trust me. One day you'll see. Trust me!"

The Lord is saying the same thing to you and me. We ask, "Why?" and He says, "Trust Me!"

WE ASK, "WHY?" AND HE SAYS "TRUST ME!"

If you can't place your faith in the Creator of the Universe, and the Giver of Life, what is the alternative? Why search anywhere else for wisdom when He *is* wisdom?

He Knows You

Remember, since God made you, He understands and knows exactly what you need. The Lord says: *"Before I formed you in the womb I knew you, before you were born I set you apart"* (Jeremiah 1:5).

69

You are not here by chance. He has called you and you're here for a purpose.

When God says, "Trust Me," don't argue with Him. If He says "jump," ask "How high?" because there'll be a blessing when your feet touch the ground.

Here are three things you must believe about God:

1. He is Omnipotent – all powerful! Not that He has some power, but *all! "I am the Lord, the God of all mankind. Is anything too hard for me?" (Jeremiah 32:27).*

2. He is Omniscient – all knowing! This means nothing can be hidden from God. *"From heaven the Lord looks down and sees all mankind"* (Psalm 33:13).

There's no point in trying to keep a secret from the Lord – He already knows it!

3. He is Omnipresent – the Lord is everywhere! *"Where can I go from your Spirit? Where can I flee from your presence?"* (Psalm 139:7). If you tell the Lord "Goodnight," it's you who is going to sleep, not Him. The Bible says He who watches over us *"will neither slumber nor sleep"* (Psalms 121:4).

I am convinced beyond a shadow of doubt there have been times when God's angels have protected me. Just as I was about to drive down a certain road or walk on a particular street, I have felt something in my spirit that warned, "Wait! Don't go there!"

It is the Lord's hand of safety covering me.

Starting Over

The major turning point of your life is the day you stop running with the world and ask God to turn your future around. When the mistakes of your past are covered with the Blood of Christ, the Lord says, "I can't even remember them." They are buried in the sea of God's forgetfulness. The Word declares, *"As far as the east is from the west, so far has he removed our transgressions from us"* (Psalms 103:12).

From that moment forward, everything changes. *"Though your sins are like scarlet, they shall be as white as snow; though they are red as crimson, they shall be like wool"* (Isaiah 1:18).

WHEN THE MISTAKES OF YOUR PAST ARE COVERED WITH THE BLOOD OF CHRIST, THE LORD SAYS, "I CAN'T EVEN REMEMBER THEM."

The reason you can become *young* again is because you've been *born* again! The Bible tells us; *"Therefore if any man be in Christ, he is a new creature: old things are passed away; behold, all things are become new"* (2 Corinthians 5:17 KJV).

This means you have a new birthday – and you're starting over as a "babe in Christ." You are changed from the inside out!

Avoid the Traps

People may not understand why, but make your decisions based on what the Lord says – not man. As a result, instead of just keeping pace with the foot soldiers, you'll start moving as fast as the chariots.

The spirit of this world is insidious – it will stifle your drive, your passion and your joy. Even more, it will stop you dead in your tracks and keep you from reaching the divine destiny God has prepared specifically for you.

THE SPIRIT OF THIS WORLD IS INSIDIOUS – IT WILL STIFLE YOUR DRIVE, YOUR PASSION AND YOUR JOY.

If you allow the devil to creep in and have his way, every desire the Lord has planted in your heart will be uprooted and discarded. The things you wanted so desperately will suddenly be out of reach.

How will Satan accomplish his desire to see you fail? He will trap you in ungodly relationships, entice you with health-destroying habits and lure you into financial failures.

Inside Out!

Most people are not destroyed from the outside in, but from the inside out!

Let me give you an example. Joy doesn't come because I share a humorous story to make you laugh. It's not the result of being in the presence of certain people – although it may help. Instead, somewhere deep within, you must be happy with yourself.

If your peace and contentment depends on another person, how will you cope if that individual is suddenly removed from your life? What will happen then?

There's something far greater that fuels my joy. I found it when I asked Jesus to forgive my sin and live in my heart. He not only gave me eternal happiness but put a smile on my face and a spring in my step. The Bible is true when it declares *"the joy of the Lord is your strength"* (Nehemiah 8:10).

IF YOUR PEACE AND CONTENTMENT DEPENDS ON ANOTHER PERSON, HOW WILL YOU COPE IF THAT INDIVIDUAL IS SUDDENLY REMOVED FROM YOUR LIFE?

I love my friends, yet if they have the power to rob me of my joy it means they are my God – and I'm not about to let that happen. The Lord says, *"I will never leave thee, nor forsake thee"* (Hebrews 13:5 KJV). He is *"a friend that sticks closer than a brother"* (Proverbs 18:24).

Your New Adventure

Will you feel a little self-conscious when your life has suddenly been changed from dull to dynamic? Of course. Every new adventure takes some adjustment. But it's a life God wants you to experience.

I'm sure Esther must have been a little uncomfortable the first time she walked into the courtroom of King Xerxes – a godless man who had no idea she was from Jewish ancestry. But every time he asked her to be with

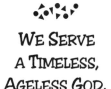

WE SERVE A TIMELESS, AGELESS GOD.

him, Esther put on her makeup and perfume, using her femininity and beauty. The Bible says, *"The girl pleased him and won his favor"* (Esther 2:9).

It was a very dangerous assignment, yet God used Esther to change the mind of a king and save a nation (Esther 9:18-23) – an event Israel celebrates to this day.

It's a Race!

We serve a timeless, ageless God. When you are 96 years old He will be the same as when you were 16. There's no point in time that escapes the presence of the Almighty. He *always* has the ability to bless you, heal you, and resurrect you.

My friend, we are not taking a slow, leisurely walk

74

through a garden of flowers, We are in a race that requires swiftness and stamina. Paul the Apostle asks, *"Do you not know that in a race all the runners run, but only one gets the prize? Run in such a way as to get the prize"* (1 Corinthians 9:24).

That is why we must, *"throw off everything that hinders and the sin that so easily entangles, and let us run with perseverance the race marked out for us"* (Hebrews 12:1).

YOU MAY BE TIRED, YET WHEN THE HAND OF THE LIVING GOD TOUCHES YOUR LIFE, YOU'LL COME ALIVE!

You may be tired, yet when the hand of the Living God touches your life, you'll come alive! The Lord will restore you. Why? Because He loves you and wants you by His side.

Jumping and Leaping!

One afternoon Peter and John were about to enter the temple when they saw a man at the gate who was crippled from birth. He was brought there every day to beg from those going into the temple courts. Peter and John said to the man "Look at us!" – and he did, expecting to receive money from them.

Then Peter continued, *"Silver or gold I do not have, but what I have I give you. In the name of Jesus Christ of*

Nazareth, walk" (Acts 3:6).

Taking him by his right hand, Peter helped the man up, and instantly the man's feet and ankles became strong. He not only jumped to his feet, the Bible records he ran into the temple courts, *"leaping, and praising God"* (v.8 KJV).

Alive Again!

The moment you put your total trust in Jehovah, two important things happen. First, He begins to move in your life. Second, you'll gain unbelievable strength. The

THINK OF IT! YOU'LL START RUNNING AND WON'T GET TIRED!

Bible tells us, *"...those who hope in the Lord will renew their strength. They will soar on wings like eagles; they will run and not grow weary, they will walk and not be faint"* (Isaiah 40:31).

Think of it! You'll start running and won't get tired!

Oh, I know what you are thinking. "If I start running I won't last long – I'll be huffing, puffing and start to feel my aches and pains."

The running we are talking about has little to do with making a 100-yard dash in ten seconds. I believe God is going to inspire you to become alive as never before:

- Your words and body language will become lively and animated.
- Your passion for life will soar.
- You'll have a sparkle in your eyes.
- You will begin to think young thoughts.

Everything about your life will be transformed – as if you've shifted gears. You will feel rejuvenated from head to toe. Just think what God is about to accomplish through you!

Put on your running shoes!

CHAPTER 5

"I'LL BE BACK!"

Without doubt, Muhammad Ali was the greatest heavyweight boxing champion ever. The man who could "float like a butterfly and sting like a bee" was a legend in his own time.

In 1964, he shocked the world by beating Sonny Liston. It was the start of a spectacular career.

However, on February 15, 1978, after a long string of title defenses, Ali lost his crown to Leon Spinks on a decision. Did that mean his career was over? Absolutely not! He grabbed the microphone and announced, "This isn't the last time you'll see me!"

Seven months later, the legendary fighter made a comeback. He beat Spinks and regained his title.

It's Not Over!

Friend, when Satan corners you and starts pounding

unmercifully, you can weather the storm since you know who's going to be the ultimate winner. He may think you're out on your feet, but you're just playing "rope-a-dope."

You see, as a believer the power you possess is that of a champion. The Word tells us: *"...greater is he that is in you, than he that is in the world"* (1 John 4:4 KJV).

EVEN IF SATAN PUMMELS YOU TO THE FLOOR, IT'S NOT OVER. WITH GOD'S HELP YOU'RE GOING TO STAND UP, KEEP FIGHTING AND GIVE THE DEVIL A TKO!

Even if Satan pummels you to the floor, it's not over. With God's help you're going to stand up, keep fighting and give the devil a TKO!

How do I know that is possible? Because the Bible clearly states: *"though a righteous man falls seven times, he rises again, but the wicked are brought down by calamity"* Proverbs 24:16).

Yes, you are going to bounce back.

Unstoppable!

Don't panic! You already know the outcome. Repeat what Arnold Schwartzenegger said in his movie, *The Terminator*: "I'll be back!"

- When you've exhausted all of your resources, say, "I'll be back!"
- When it seems all hope is gone, say, "I'll be back!"
- When you stumble and fall, say, "I'll be back!"
- When others believe you are finished, say "I'll be back!"

The journey doesn't end until God says so. That's why you can view every setback as temporary.

The Almighty commands you: *"Take up your positions; stand firm and see the deliverance the Lord will give you...Do not be afraid; do not be discouraged...the Lord will be with you"* (2 Chronicles 20:17).

THE JOURNEY DOESN'T END UNTIL GOD SAYS SO. THAT'S WHY YOU CAN VIEW EVERY SETBACK AS TEMPORARY.

Excuses! Excuses!

I can still remember a woman who only occasionally came to our church telling me, "I'm tired of serving the Lord."

"Serving the Lord? I asked her. "How many times do you attend church each month?"

"Oh, once or twice," she responded.

I couldn't believe my ears. Here was a woman complaining of being tired and "suffering for Jesus," yet she was hardly involved in the Body of Christ.

Some people will use any flimsy excuse to justify staying away from God's house:

- "It rained this morning and ruined my hair."
- "I had a bad week at the office and I need to relax and take time for myself!"
- "They don't sing the hymns I like."
- "Sometimes I feel closer to God when I'm out on a lake fishing."

Since one excuse is as good as another, you may as well say, "I'm not going to church this week because I'm out of chocolate milk!"

The Blood of Martyrs

THE MAJORITY OF CHRISTIANS IN AMERICA HAVE NO CONCEPT OF WHAT IT MEANS TO SUFFER FOR THE CAUSE OF CHRIST.

The majority of Christians in America have no concept of what it means to suffer for the cause of Christ. They don't understand that people around the world have literally shed their blood to serve Jesus.

My family escaped to

America because of the religious persecution in their homeland – Armenia.

In 1915 – and the tragic years that followed – the Turks annihilated nearly 2 million Christian Armenians. Entire cities were wiped off the map. Torture, pillage, rape and murder spread unchecked across the land.

Why? Because people chose to stand up for their faith in Christ. The massacres were beyond human imagination. Those people didn't just give lip service to being a Christian; they gave their lives!

Even today, the blood of these Armenian martyrs cries out, urging us to live for Jesus – regardless of the cost. I am proud to be part of that heritage.

The Secret

Throughout history, many who have declared their allegiance to the Living God have paid a high price.

In the Old Testament you will read the story of Samson, a mighty warrior who was feared by the Philistines. When he fell in love with a woman named Delilah, the rulers of the Philistines went to her and said, *"See if you can lure him into showing you the secret of his great strength and how we can overpower him so we may tie him up and subdue him. Each one of us will give you eleven hundred shekels of silver"* (Judges 16:5).

One night, when Samson was extremely tired, he revealed his secret, telling Delilah, *"No razor has ever been used on my head...because I have been a Nazirite set apart to God since birth. If my head were shaved, my strength would leave me, and I would become as weak as any other man"* (v.17).

"IF MY HEAD WERE SHAVED, MY STRENGTH WOULD LEAVE ME, AND I WOULD BECOME AS WEAK AS ANY OTHER MAN."
— JUDGES 16:17

Immediately, she sent word to the rulers of the Philistines, and while Samson was sleeping on her lap, a man shaved his head and he was subdued. The covenant God made with Samson had been broken.

They seized him, gouged out his eyes, and threw him in prison where he was forced to spend his days grinding grain.

The People Laughed

With their foe imprisoned, the people began to celebrate. The Bible records that *"While they were in high spirits, they shouted, 'Bring out Samson to entertain us.'"* (v.25).

They didn't notice that Samson's hair was beginning to grow back.

Now blind, the prisoner was brought to the temple, where all the people could mock and ridicule him. He said to the servant who guided his hands, *"Put me where I can feel the pillars that support the temple, so that I may lean against them"* (v.26).

Here was God's champion – and the throngs were laughing at him. The Bible says about 3,000 people were present (v.27) and Samson was the joke of the day!

Strong Again!

Samson prayed to the Lord: *"O Sovereign Lord, remember me. O God, please strengthen me just once more, and let me with one blow get revenge on the Philistines for my two eyes"* (v.28).

❖•❖•❖•

IN HIS SPIRIT, SAMSON WAS SAYING, "I MAY BE BLIND, BUT I'LL BE BACK!"

He wasn't upset at Delilah's betrayal or his unwanted haircut, rather that his sight was gone. In his spirit, Samson was saying, "I may be blind, but I'll be back!"

Then he reached toward the two central pillars on which the temple stood. *"Bracing himself against them, his right hand on the one and his left hand on the other,*

85

Samson said, 'Let me die with the Philistines!'" (vv.29-30).

Pushing with all his might, *"down came the temple on the rulers and all the people in it. Thus he killed many more when he died than while he lived"* (v.30).

Samson's strength returned – and he brought the house down!

"All Things!"

People may have belittled you for serving God, yet you can declare, "In the Name of Jesus I'm going to be what the Lord has called me to be. I'm not going to give up!"

YOU CAN DECLARE, "IN THE NAME OF JESUS, I'M GOING TO BE WHAT THE LORD HAS CALLED ME TO BE. I'M NOT GOING TO GIVE UP!"

Why allow the devil to stop Jehovah's power in your life? Yes, you will have setbacks and discouragement, yet God is still God.

Remember, you can do *"all things"* through Christ who strengthens you (Philippians 4:13). When you are weak, He gives you the power to bounce back!

A Remarkable Comeback

Even if you have experienced a financial reversal, it's

not the end of the world. In 1990, Donald Trump, one of New York's real estate tycoons, suddenly found himself on the skids. His empire crumbled when he was forced into bankruptcy with over $2 billion in bank loans he couldn't pay.

But ever the dealmaker, he engineered one of the most remarkable rebounds in business history.

In his book, *The Art of the Comeback,* Trump says that being fervent about what you do is a key ingredient to rising from the ashes. He offers this advice: "If you don't have passion about who you are, about what you are trying to be, about where you are going, you might as well give up. Passion is the essence of life, and certainly the essence of success."

"PASSION IS THE ESSENCE OF LIFE, AND CERTAINLY THE ESSENCE OF SUCCESS."
— DONALD TRUMP

By the year 2000 Donald Trump was again worth over one billion dollars.

Extraordinary!

Some people pray for an apple, then pout like a child when they can't have it immediately. They don't realize that God is trying to give them an entire orchard!

We don't serve a "half-way" Lord.

Attending a wedding at Cana in Galilee, Jesus' mother told Him, "They have no more wine."

Nearby there were six stone water jars, the type used by the Jews for ceremonial washing, each holding from twenty to thirty gallons. Jesus said to the servants, *"'Fill the jars with water'; so they filled them to the brim"* (John 2:7).

Jesus Doesn't Do Anything "Average"- Only the Best! Just as He Did With the Wine, He Takes Ordinary People and Makes them Extraordinary.

Then He told them to draw some out and take it to the master of the banquet. When they did, the man *"tasted the water that had been turned into wine. He did not realize where it had come from, though the servants who had drawn the water knew"* (v.9).

The master of the banquet called the bridegroom aside and commented: *"Everyone brings out the choice wine first and then the cheaper wine after the guests have had too much to drink; but you have saved the best till now"* (v.10).

Jesus doesn't do anything "average" – only the *best!* Just as He did with the wine, He takes ordinary people and makes them extraordinary.

A King in a Cave

When everything in your life seems black and people are telling you it's over, say with David, *"You are my lamp, O Lord; the Lord turns my darkness into light"* (2 Samuel 22:29).

Think of all the problems David endured. After being anointed king over Israel, Saul became so jealous that David had to flee into the wilderness for fourteen years because of a death threat that was made on his life.

Hiding in a cave, the Lord was still assuring David, "Yes, you are a king – even if you happen to be in this horrible place. One day the world will know!"

Despite the mistake David made with Bathsheba, God saw the repentance in his heart and forgave him. David later wrote: *"I acknowledged my sin to you and did not cover up my iniquity. I said, 'I will confess my transgressions to the Lord' – and you forgave the guilt of my sin"* (Psalm 32:5).

"I ACKNOWLEDGED MY SIN TO YOU AND DID NOT COVER UP MY INIQUITY. I SAID, 'I WILL CONFESS MY TRANSGRESSIONS TO THE LORD' – AND YOU FORGAVE THE GUILT OF MY SIN."
- PSALM 32:5

Bitter Soldiers

Once, when David and his army were involved in one of their conquests, the Amalikites descended on the camp where the families of the Israeli soldiers were living. The enemy not only stole all their goods and set the place on fire, but *"their wives, and their sons, and their daughters, were taken captives"* (1 Samuel 30:3).

It was such a tragedy that *"David and the people that were with him lifted up their voice and wept, until they had no more power to weep"* (v.4).

DAVID'S SOLDIER'S WERE NO LONGER EXALTING HIM, SAYING, "OH, MIGHTY KING. YOU'RE THE ONE WHO DEFEATED THE GIANT!"

At this point, David's soldiers were no longer exalting him, saying, "Oh, mighty King. You're the one who defeated the giant!" They did not dance and sing, *"Saul has slain his thousands, and David his tens of thousands"* (1 Samuel 18:7).

Far from it! David was greatly distressed *"because the men were talking of stoning him; each one was bitter in spirit because of his sons and daughters"* (1 Samuel 30:6).

Total Recovery

How did David react? Since his troops had turned on

him, and his family had been taken hostage, he was all alone. Yet, David had the one true friend he needed. The Bible says, *"David encouraged himself in the Lord his God"* (1 Samuel 30:6).

Upset with the enemy, He thought, "You may have taken our wives, our children and our belongings, but we'll be back!"

To the troops he ordered, "Saddle up the horses!" – and they invaded the city where the women and children were held captive.

Scripture records: *"David recovered everything the Amalekites had taken... Nothing was missing: young or old, boy or girl, plunder or anything else they had taken. David brought everything back"* (vv.18-19).

What a victory!

I can only imagine what the outcome would have been had David agreed with his troops and admitted, "You're right! I'm a low-down, good-for-nothing king. Go ahead and kill me!"

Like David, there are times you need to get away from the negatives and hear only from God. Let Him

I CAN ONLY IMAGINE WHAT THE OUTCOME WOULD HAVE BEEN HAD DAVID AGREED WITH HIS TROOPS AND ADMITTED, "YOU'RE RIGHT! I'M A LOW-DOWN, GOOD-FOR-NOTHING KING. GO AHEAD AND KILL ME!"

give you a pep-talk, encouraging you to: "Stand to your feet and get back in the fight!" He is you Captain and you will prevail!

David's Rock

From personal experience, David could state: *"As for God, his way is perfect; the word of the Lord is tried: he is a buckler to all them that trust in him"* (2 Samuel 22:31 KJV). Your Father is the one who supports you when you are carrying a heavy load.

NEVER ALLOW THE DEVIL TO DICTATE YOUR FUTURE. HE'S NOT THE ONE WHO DETERMINES THE HEALTH AND HAPPINESS YOU ARE GOING TO ENJOY.

The Lord was David's Rock – the strength and power he needed to renew his youth and start over. That's why he was able to exclaim: *"He makes my feet like the feet of a deer; he enables me to stand on the heights"* (2 Samuel 22:34).

God will totally restore and recharge your life – providing you with everything necessary to reach the summit.

"Wait a Minute!"

Never allow the devil to dictate your future. He's not the one who determines the health and happiness you are going to enjoy.

The moment Satan tries to infiltrate your life, resist him and say: "Wait a minute! You are ignorant – without wisdom! You had know idea what you were doing when you declared war on God. How can you tell me how to live when you're a miserable failure?"

Let the devil know you are going to trust the true and living God – and that you plan to walk in the power of the Holy Spirit.

One More Try

Of course, there will be tough times – but you serve a tough God! When everything around you seems to be collapsing, He is by your side.

Don't limit the power of God in your life. Regardless of the past, you can begin once more and achieve victories beyond your greatest dreams. You can exclaim: *"...for I know whom I have believed, and am persuaded that he is able to keep that which I have committed unto him against that day"* (2 Timothy 1:12 KJV).

> DON'T LIMIT THE POWER OF GOD IN YOUR LIFE. REGARDLESS OF THE PAST, YOU CAN BEGIN ONCE MORE AND ACHIEVE VICTORIES BEYOND YOUR GREATEST DREAMS.

Our God is able to turn darkness into light.

The Third Day!

Every Christian knows what took place at the crucifixion of Christ. It was on a crude, wooden Cross that Jesus shed His precious Blood as a substitute for the sins of man – so that you and I could receive salvation.

THE DAY OF OUR GREATEST CELEBRATION IS NOT WHAT HAPPENED AT CALVARY, BUT THE MIRACULOUS EVENT AT THE GARDEN TOMB THREE DAYS LATER – THE RESURRECTION.

However, the day of our greatest celebration is not what happened at Calvary, but the miraculous event at the garden tomb three days later – the resurrection.

If people had only listened to the words of Jesus before He died, they would not have been so surprised when He rose from the grave. More than once, Christ explained to His disciples that *"he must go to Jerusalem and suffer many things at the hands of the elders, chief priests and teachers of the law, and that he must be killed and on the third day be raised to life"* (Matthew 16:21).

Jesus was telling them, "I must complete the purpose for which I was sent to earth. Yes, I will die on the Cross, but don't worry, I'll be back!"

It was Friday – but Sunday was coming!

What a Shock!

The body of Jesus had been wrapped in linen and placed in a borrowed tomb. Then, on the first day of the week, very early in the morning, the women from Galilee took some spices they had prepared and went to the tomb.

JESUS WAS TELLING THEM, "I MUST COMPLETE THE PURPOSE FOR WHICH I WAS SENT TO EARTH. YES, I WILL DIE ON THE CROSS, BUT DON'T WORRY, I'LL BE BACK!"

What a shock that must have been!" As Scripture records: *They found the stone rolled away from the tomb, but when they entered, they did not find the body of the Lord Jesus* (Luke 24:2-3).

In the midst of their amazement, suddenly two men in clothes that gleamed like lightning stood beside them. Frightened, the women bowed down with their faces to the ground, and the men said to them, *"Why do you look for the living among the dead? He is not here; he has risen! Remember how he told you, while he was still with you in Galilee: 'The Son of Man must be delivered into the hands of sinful men, be crucified and on the third day be raised again.' Then they remembered his words"* (vv.5-8).

Jesus had previously announced, "I'll be back!" – and, Hallelujah, He kept His word.

"I Will Come Again"

After the resurrection, Jesus appeared to Mary Magdalene and the women at the tomb, to two travelers on the road to Emamaus, to the disciples, and *"to more than five hundred"* (1 Corinthians 15:6).

Now He had a new message. As part of God's divine plan, He told them He was going back to heaven, but would not forget about them. He promised to return.

AGAIN AND AGAIN, THE SON OF GOD PROMISED, "I AM GOING AWAY AND I AM COMING BACK TO YOU."
- JOHN 14:28

Jesus said to the disciples, *"...if I go and prepare a place for you, I will come again, and receive you unto myself; that where I am, there ye may be also"* (John 14:3 KJV).

Again and again, the Son of God promised, *"I am going away and I am coming back to you."* (John 14:28).

If you know Christ as your Lord and Savior, He will be returning for you, *"For the Son of Man is going to come in his Father's glory with his angels, and then he will reward each person according to what he has done"* (Matthew 16:27).

Today, the Lord is saying: "Love Me, live for Me, and get ready for that great day. I'll be back!"

CHAPTER 6

TAKE IT
TO THE LIMIT
ONE MORE TIME

There were often tears in my grandfather's eyes when he was a youngster. He looked across the fields, watching kids going off to school in South Georgia. Instead – with only a third-grade education – he was plowing the land, helping to support the family.

Inside that young man, however, was a burning passion to expand his boundaries; to live to the fullest. That's exactly what he did! Before he left this earth for his heavenly reward, my grandfather (on my mom's side) became one of the esteemed leaders of his church denomination, and sat with kings and presidents.

Rather than remaining on that dusty field, he created a new one – and sowed precious seed into the lives of untold thousands!

Holy Boldness!

My Armenian grandfather – on my dad's side – also left an indelible mark on this world. In every aspect of his life, he was as bold as a lion.

IN EVERY ASPECT OF HIS LIFE, HE WAS AS BOLD AS A LION.

When some men broke into his home in Los Angeles they quickly learned they had made a big mistake. The house was a "shotgun" design – with one door in the front, another in the back, and a long hall connecting the rooms. Grandpa ran to the back door, but instead of leaving, he locked it!

"What in the world are you doing?" one of the intruders asked.

Rushing to the front door and doing the same thing, he shouted, "I'm locking you in!" Then he proceeded to clobber those thieves senseless.

He threw those frightened rascals out of the house and they never returned!

"How Dare You!"

Grandpa fought the devil with the same ferocity. Once, when he was working on an Army base in

Arizona, the entire region was in the midst of a severe drought.

One afternoon, while trying to repair some air conditioning units, he heard a man cursing God because of the lack of rain!"

Speaking in broken English, he said, "Mister, you can't talk to God like that. Why are you using such language?

"Because it's His #@% fault this land is so dry!"

Right on the spot, my grandfather responded, "Well, sir, I believe in God and I'm not going to curse Him. Instead, I am going to pray. And by noon tomorrow it's going to rain!"

"MISTER, YOU CAN'T TALK TO GOD LIKE THAT. WHY ARE YOU USING SUCH LANGUAGE?"

Word quickly spread like wildfire, and the people on the Army base thought my grandfather was crazy.

Where's the Rain?

What happened next sounds incredible, but many have verified the story.

The following day, about 11:45 A.M. – fifteen minutes before he prophesied it would rain – my grandpa put on his swimming trunks and walked outside of his house on the Army base in the middle of that desert.

They were now *positive* he was nuts! And the neighbors started to jeer. "Look at you!" they laughed, "There's not a cloud in the sky!"

Suddenly, five minutes before noon, the heavens darkened and there was a crack of thunder. Then bolts of lightning began hitting the ground. It didn't just sprinkle – there was a torrential downpour that flooded the parched earth. And there was grandpa, dancing around in his swim trunks!

THERE IS NO SUPPRESSING A MAN OR WOMAN WHO BELIEVES GOD CAN CHANGE EVERY CIRCUMSTANCE.

In the years that followed, God graced him with an effective ministry around the world.

I am reminded of both my grandfathers every time a radio station plays the Eagles' hit song of the 1970s, "Take it to the Limit One More Time!"

That's exactly what they practiced!

There is no suppressing a man or woman who believes God can change every circumstance.

"Get Out!"

Jesus wasn't timid.

Once, when it was almost time for the Jewish Passover, Jesus traveled to Jerusalem. In the temple courts He was shocked to see men selling livestock, and others exchanging money.

Scripture records that He *"made a whip out of cords, and drove all from the temple area, both sheep and cattle; he scattered the coins of the money changers and overturned their tables"* (John 2:15).

Jesus demanded, *"Get these out of here! How dare you turn my Father's house into a market!"* (v.16).

His actions often upset the religious leaders of the day.

When the Lord healed the paralytic at the pool of Bethesda, the Jewish leaders were offended because He was doing these things on the Sabbath.

"MY FATHER IS ALWAYS AT HIS WORK TO THIS VERY DAY, AND I, TOO, AM WORKING."
- JOHN 5:17

Jesus didn't hesitate to tell them: *"My Father is always at his work to this very day, and I, too, am working"* (John 5:17).

He pushed the scribes and Pharisees to the limit.

"Do You Believe?"

In Capernaum, two blind men followed Jesus, calling out, *"Have mercy on us, Son of David!"* (Matthew 9:27).

Jesus asked an important question: *"Do you believe that I am able to do this?"* (v.28).

"Yes, Lord" they replied.

Immediately, He touched their eyes and said: *"According to your faith will it be done to you"* (v.29) – and their sight was restored.

What is the Lord looking for? Faith!

"He's Calling You!"

At the ancient city of Jericho, about 15 miles northeast of Jerusalem, Jesus and the disciples attracted a large crowd. As they were leaving, a blind man was sitting by the side of the road, begging. His name was Bartimaeus.

Hearing it was Jesus of Nazareth, he began to shout, *"Jesus, Son of David, have mercy on me!"* (Mark 10:47).

WHAT IS THE LORD LOOKING FOR? FAITH! Many rebuked the beggar telling him to be quiet, but Bartimaeus shouted even louder: *"Son of David, have mercy on me!"* (v.48).

The Bible records that Jesus stopped, looked at the man and said, *"Call him."* (v.49).

So they called to the blind man, *"Cheer up! On your feet! He's calling you"* (v.49).

Bartimaeus threw his cloak aside, jumped up and came to the Lord.

"What do you want me to do for you?" Jesus asked him.

The blind man answered, "Rabbi, I want to see."

*"'Go,' said Jesus, 'your faith has healed you.'
Immediately he received his sight and followed Jesus
along the road"* (v.52).

An "Impossible" Proposal

Oh, what a difference it makes when you walk by faith, and not by sight!

I have learned that when you reach the point of no return, God is patiently waiting! In response to your belief, He is there.

As I look back on our ministry in Atlanta, Georgia, we were always stretching ourselves to the limit – time after time.

With a small congregation and $300 in the bank, the Lord showed me 23 acres of land and gave me a vision to expand the ministry. He said, "This is where I want you to build the church."

> WHAT A
> DIFFERENCE IT
> MAKES WHEN YOU
> WALK BY FAITH, AND
> NOT BY SIGHT!

I told our congregation, "If God said it, we can do it!"

Some people laughed, yet I believed with all my heart a marvelous work for the Lord would be built on that property.

I told my dream to the executive officers of a local bank and they though it was just that – a dream. We had neither the collateral or the track record to launch into a major project.

Well, I found out later, the board of that bank talked and talked about my "impossible" proposal. Then one day they talked themselves into giving us a startup loan of $1 million. When that decision was being made, one of the officers exclaimed (and this is exactly how he said it): "You mean we're going to loan a million dollars to a damn inspiration!"

WHEN THE LORD SAYS IT AND YOU HAVE THE FAITH TO BELIEVE, EVERYTHING IS POSSIBLE!

It was an inspiration that God abundantly blessed. You see, when the Lord says it and you have the faith to believe, *everything* is possible!

A Man of Passion

Jesus was both God and man. He was *"in very nature God...made in human likeness"* (Philippians 2:6-7). His name was Immanuel – which means, *"God with us"* (Matthew 1:23).

Christ was also a Man of passion:

- A passion to do the will of His Father: *"For I have come down from heaven not to do my will but to do the will of him who sent me"* (John 6:38).

- A passion to redeem sinners: *"For the Son of Man came to seek and to save what was lost"* (Luke 19:10).
- A passion to defeat Satan: *"The reason the Son of God appeared was to destroy the devil's work* (1 John 3:8).
- A passion to complete His destiny: *"Father, into your hands I commit my spirit"* (Luke 23:46).

The Lord not only offers passion, but *com*passion – especially for those who experience a limited existence. He states: *"I am come that they might have life, and that they might have it more abundantly"* (John 10:10 KJV).

"THE REASON THE SON OF GOD APPEARED WAS TO DESTROY THE DEVIL'S WORK."

- 1 JOHN 3:8

Oh, the Suffering

Personally, Jesus took His flesh to the limit, so we could have eternal life. Critics of Mel Gibson's motion picture, *The Passion of the Christ,* say, "I don't understand why they had to portray so much violence, so much bloodshed."

So much? I believe the film gives us only a small

glimpse of the pain and torture Jesus suffered for you and me.

Crucifixion was a practice that originated with the Persians, but the Romans perfected it as a method of capital punishment to cause maximum pain and suffering over a significant period of time – far longer than the two hours of Gibson's film.

IT IS ALMOST IMPOSSIBLE TO COMPREHEND THE MAGNITUDE OF WHAT THE SAVIOR ENDURED.

Through the prophet Isaiah, the Lord said, *"I offered my back to those who beat me, my cheeks to those who pulled out my beard; I did not hide my face from mocking and spitting"* (Isaiah 50:6).

In the movie, even after the many beatings, we could still recognize the face of Jesus. However, in reality, it was far worse. The Bible says, many were *"appalled at him – his appearance was so disfigured beyond that of any man and his form marred beyond human likeness"* (Isaiah 52:14).

Great Drops of Blood

It is almost impossible to comprehend the magnitude of what the Savior endured at Calvary. *"They spit on him, and took the staff and struck him on the head again and again"* (Matthew 27:30).

The scourging continued. *"And being in anguish, he prayed more earnestly, and his sweat was like drops of blood falling to the ground"* (Luke 22:44).

Medical doctors who have studied the crucifixion say His body literally exploded – burst open.

Jesus was brutally punished for no *crime* that He had committed, yet the Father permitted the Cross so that you and I can find salvation.

"Forgive Them"

At Calvary, Jesus took love and mercy to the limit. *"Having loved his own who were in the world, he now showed them the full extent of his love"* (John 13:1).

In the natural He would have hated and reviled those who were cursing and spitting upon Him. Yet, on the Cross, Jesus looked toward heaven and said, *"Father, forgive them, for they do not know what they are doing"* (Luke 23:34).

HIS HANDS REACHED OUT TO HEAL AND HELP, YET THEY WERE NAILED TO A CROSS.

His hands reached out to *heal and help*, yet they were nailed to a Cross.

Christ defined the word *endurance* for our redemption. That's why we must *"fix our eyes on Jesus, the author and perfecter of our faith, who for the joy set before him endured the cross, scorning its shame, and sat down at the right hand of the throne of God"* (Hebrews 12:2).

Limitless Power

What an example Jesus gave us. He went farther than any man to clear the path for you and me. Why? Because when we reach our point of no return we can say, "The Lord has already been here! He is with me right now!"

BECAUSE OF THE CROSS, THE SAME LIMITLESS POWER OF GOD THAT WAS IN JESUS RESIDES IN YOU AND ME.

In the Garden of Gethsemane His flesh cried out, *"Father, if you are willing, take this cup from me; yet not my will, but yours be done"* (Luke 22:42).

Because of the Cross, the same limitless power of God that was in Jesus resides in you and me. If He overcame the world, the flesh and the devil, so can we!

Don't listen to the carnal man who keeps reminding you how weak and sinful you are. Satan longs to hear you cry, "I'm at the end of my rope. I am not going to make it."

Jesus ascended to heaven, but He sent the Holy Spirit to be our Teacher, Comforter and Guide. As a result, you are not walking this road alone. He says: *"Never will I leave you; never will I forsake you"* (Hebrews 13:5).

It's For Today

I remember talking with a woman who was totally distraught over the circumstances of her life.

"Have you accepted Christ as your Savior?" I asked her.

"Yes, I have," she replied.

"Then where do you think you will spend eternity?"

"I know I'm going to heaven," she confidently stated.

Switching the topic back to her immediate problem, I continued, "If you believe God is preparing your eternal resting place, why don't you have faith that the Lord can bless you here on earth?"

> THE SAME LORD WHO WANTS TO BUILD YOU A HOME IN THE BY-AND -BY, IS READY TO GIVE YOU UNLIMITED PROVISION IN THE HERE-AND-NOW!

The same Lord who wants to build you a home in the by-and-by, is ready to give you unlimited provision in the here-and-now! Why? Because He desires to demonstrate to the world how much He loves His children.

The Overcomers

When you fully realize what Christ has done, you'll

begin to rise from defeat and depression. You will find reasons to live!

Jesus came in the flesh so that we could walk in the spirit. He took His flesh to the limit, so we wouldn't be limited in our flesh. As a result, we can have power to overcome every hurdle.

JESUS CAME IN THE FLESH SO THAT WE COULD WALK IN THE SPIRIT.

It's one thing to have strength and ability, but Christ moves us to a new level – *overcoming* power.

This means when you run up against one of life's obstacles, you don't beat your head against the wall – you leap *over* it!

Here are three vital principles:

1. Because you have asked Christ to come into your heart, you are an overcomer. For *"everyone born of God overcomes the world"* (1 John 5:4).

2. Your power comes directly from the Lord. He says, *"I have given you authority to trample on snakes and scorpions and to overcome all the power of the enemy"* (Luke 10:19).

3. You have the power to defeat Satan. *"You, dear children, are from God and have overcome them, because the one who is in you is greater than the one who* *is in the world"* (1 John 4:4).

No one is holding your feet to the ground. Take a step of faith and move from the visible to the invisible – into God's Spirit. As Paul wrote: *"So we fix our eyes not on what is seen, but on what is unseen. For what is seen is temporary, but what is unseen is eternal"* (2 Corinthians 4:18).

Why do we need overcoming power? After salvation, it is your key to eternity. The Lord promises: *"To him who overcomes, I will give the right to sit with me on my throne, just as I overcame and sat down with my Father on his throne"* (Revelation 3:21).

TAKE A STEP OF FAITH AND MOVE FROM THE VISIBLE INTO THE INVISIBLE.

Start Pulling!

Most people miss what the Lord has prepared for them because they believe, "If I can't see it, I can't have it." That is not faith.

Prayerfully and aggressively, you have to move into areas that may be unclear. Reach in and say:

- ■ "I *need* that new job" – and by faith pull that job *out!*

- "I *desire* that new relationship," and by faith pull that relationship out!
- "I *claim* my healing through Christ" – and by faith pull that healing out!

SOMEWHERE, SOMETIME, YOU MUST EXERT SOME ENERGY: GET UP, GET OUT, AND GET GOING!

Some people stand before a closed door and complain, "I'll never get it open!" when all they need to do is simply turn the doorknob.

Others moan, "I am not sure how I'm going to climb those stairs." Don't they know they have to lift their feet and move higher one step at a time?

Get Going!

One man told me, "I've been looking for a new job."

"Where are you looking?" I asked him.

His answer blew me away. He replied, "I've been praying in my bedroom."

I politely reminded him that *"faith without works is dead"* (James 2:26).

Somewhere, sometime you must exert some energy: get up, get out, and get going!

Don't sell yourself short.

I know people who lacked experience, had a limited

education and yet they landed a good job. How is that possible?

Here's the secret. Because of their relationship with the Lord, these individuals were so filled with faith, confidence and enthusiasm, the person who hired them saw their potential. In one case, the boss exclaimed, "We really don't have an opening, but we're going to make one for a person like you!"

An Investment?

Recently I was having a conversation with a young man who remarked, "I really believe I'm going to make it big this year in investments."

"Well, how much have you put into the market?" I asked him.

"Nothing," he replied. "I'm afraid I might lose it –

"IF YOU EXPECT ANY KIND OF A RETURN, YOU'VE GOT TO TAKE A STEP OF FAITH."

but I believe God is going to bring a great opportunity my way."

I hated to disappoint him, but felt it was my duty to explain, "That's not the way it works. If you expect any kind of a return, you've got to take a step of faith."

Who Can You Trust?

Jesus tells a story concerning a man who was going

on a journey. He called his three servants together and entrusted his property to them. To the first he gave five talents of money (a talent was worth more than a thousand dollars). The second servant received two talents, and the third was given just one talent.

Then the man went on his journey.

Here's what happened. *"The man who had received the five talents went at once and put his money to work and gained five more. So also, the one with the two talents gained two more. But the man who had received the one talent went off, dug a hole in the ground and hid his master's money"* (Matthew 25:16-18).

After considerable time, the master returned home and settled the accounts with his servants. The man who was entrusted with five talents gained five more. And the servant who was given two talents also doubled the value.

Don't Hide It!

To each of these wise investors, the master smiled and said, *"Well done, good and faithful servant! You have been faithful with a few things; I will put you in charge of many things. Come and share your master's happiness!"* (v.23).

Then came the man who had received the one talent. He look at the master and said, *"I knew that you are a hard man, harvesting where you have not sown and gathering where you have not scattered seed. So I was afraid and went out and hid your talent in the ground. See, here is what belongs to you"* (vv.24-25).

The master was upset, and replied: *"You wicked, lazy servant!...Well then, you should have put my money on deposit with the bankers, so that when I returned I would have received it back with interest"* (vv.26-27).

IF YOU EXPECT A GREAT RETURN, YOU HAVE TO LAUNCH OUT IN FAITH!

He took the money back and gave it to the one who had the ten talents.

The heart of the story is that if you expect a great return, you have to launch out in faith!

To the Max!

Your Heavenly Father risked everything for you, why not do the same for Him?

Go ahead and push forward with all your might. Then, when you feel you've reached your capacity, let the Lord take over – for *"God gives the Spirit without limit"* (John 3:34).

One more time, flex your faith to the max! Then stand back and watch what the Living God will do.

CHAPTER 7

AIN'T GOING DOWN 'TIL THE SUN COMES UP!

Do you know what it's like to spend your nights tossing and turning – crying instead of sleeping? Have there been times when you were so filled with anxiety and worry that your eyes never closed?

Don't feel alone. If you read the book of Psalms, you'll discover that David shared your experience. He cried out to God, *"Be merciful to me, Lord, for I am faint; O Lord, heal me, for my bones are in agony. My soul is in anguish. How long, O Lord, how long? Turn, O Lord, and deliver me; save me because of your unfailing love. No one remembers you when he is dead. Who praises you from the grave? I am worn out from groaning; all night long I flood my bed with weeping and drench my couch with tears. My eyes grow weak with sorrow; they fail because of all my foes"* (Psalm 6:2-7).

That's a first-class job of complaining!

Your Escape

David's story, however, doesn't end in bitter tears. He found the way *out* of life's troubling storms. Keep reading the Book of Psalms and you will follow the path to his ultimate victory. He exclaimed, *"I waited patiently for the Lord; he turned to me and heard my cry"* (Psalm 40:1). That's why he could exclaim: *"Let God arise, let his enemies be scattered"* (Psalm 68:1 KJV).

REGARDLESS OF THE UPHEAVAL YOU MAY BE EXPERIENCING, HELP AND HOPE IS CLOSER THAN YOU REALIZE.

Perhaps at this very moment – as you are reading this book – your life is in turmoil and your emotions are frayed:

- A trusted friend has betrayed you.
- Your career is in jeopardy.
- The doctor has given you a negative report.
- A member of your family is in crisis.

Regardless of the upheaval you may be experiencing, help and hope is closer than you realize. The Lord is with you in the midnight hour and, like David, you will one day be able to tell the world: *"...weeping may remain for a night, but rejoicing comes in the morning"* (Psalm 30:5).

Country singer Garth Brooks expressed it another way: "Ain't Going Down 'Til the Sun Comes Up!"

"Arise, Shine"

Your situation may seem darker than a moonless night, yet I believe if you will put the principles we've been sharing into practice, your world will be radiantly transformed. Your Father is saying: *Arise, shine, for your light has come, and the glory of the Lord rises upon you"* (Isaiah 60:1).

Say "goodbye" to despondency and despair. Morning has broken and it's a brand new day. *"See, darkness covers the earth and thick darkness is over the peoples, but the Lord rises upon you and his glory appears over you"* (Isaiah 60:2).

STOP MOANING, "I'M TIRED," AND REALIZE YOU SERVE AN ALL-POWERFUL LORD.

It's time for the redeemed of the Lord to walk in the power and might of the Holy Spirit – to put down that defeated spirit and take their rightful place as priests of God.

Stop moaning, "I'm tired," and realize you serve an all-powerful Lord. The Word tells you to *"Beat your plowshares into swords and your pruning hooks into spears. Let the weakling say, 'I am strong!'"* (Joel 3:10).

Dynamite!

You may resemble the farmer who has plowed the same ground over and over until *he* feels like dirt. The Lord is telling you through His Word to take what you have and turn it into an instrument of spiritual warfare. He says,"Take courage and fight the good fight of faith!"

The Spirit of the Almighty is resting on you and nothing is impossible!

THE LORD WILL GIVE YOU MIRACULOUS POWER TO PREVAIL - SOMETHING BEYOND THE NATURAL.

When you are weak, God will give you the *dunamis* to prevail. That's the Greek word for *power* and *force* – from which we derive our word *dynamite!*

The Lord will give you *miraculous power* to prevail – something beyond the natural. Along with it, you'll receive the ability and the abundance that only the Father can bestow.

It's Close!

It may surprise you to know that perhaps you already *possess* your miracle.

After the Lord told Moses to lead the children of Israel out of Egypt, he became concerned and asked God, *"What if they do not believe me or listen to me and say, 'The Lord did not appear to you'?"* (Exodus 4:1).

God said to him: *"What is that in your hand?"* (v.2). "A staff," he replied.(Exodus 4:2).

You see, the Lord was about to use something Moses already owned!

God instructed him to throw the rod on the ground – and when he did, *"it became a snake, and he ran from it"* (v.3).

Then the Lord said, *"'Reach out your hand and take it by the tail.' So Moses reached out and took hold of the snake and it turned back into a staff in his hand"* (v.4).

What was the purpose of this miracle? It was *"so that they may believe that the Lord, the God of their fathers – the God of Abraham, the God of Isaac and the God of Jacob – has appeared to you"* (Exodus 4:5).

Don't worry Moses! The Lord has a plan.

CERTAINLY, THERE'S A TIME TO PRAY, BUT THERE IS ALSO A MOMENT WHEN YOU MUST TAKE ACTION AND MOVE FORWARD.

"Let God Arise!"

Certainly, there's a time to pray, but there is also a moment when you must take action and move forward. Every morning, when you see the sun welcoming the day, say, "Thank You Lord, I feel You arising within me!"

- When fear has you in its grip, let God arise!
- When evil surrounds you, let God arise!
- When perplexing problems confound you, let God arise!

Believe me, the One who created everything knows how to deal with the issue you face – and has the solution to your dilemma. Say with the psalmist, *"The Lord is my light and my salvation; whom shall I fear? The Lord is the strength of my life; of whom shall I be afraid? When evil men advance against me to devour my flesh, when my enemies and my foes attack me, they will stumble and fall"* (Psalm 27:1-2).

WHEN PERPLEXING PROBLEMS CONFOUND YOU, LET GOD ARISE!

He was not only giving himself a pep-talk, David was affirming that God was his Protector and Defender. As a result, he was filled with this assurance: *"Though an army besiege me, my heart will not fear; though war break out against me, even then will I be confident"* (v.3).

Let go and let God! Relax in His promises.

The Ultimate Shelter

David was a mighty warrior, yet waging war on a

field of battle was not his over-riding desire. Here is what he truly longed for: *"One thing I ask of the Lord, this is what I seek: that I may dwell in the house of the Lord all the days of my life, to gaze upon the beauty of the Lord and to seek him in his temple"* (v.4).

God's house is the ultimate shelter – a divine place that cannot be pierced by Satan's arrows. As David confirms: *"For in the day of trouble he will keep me safe in his dwelling; he will hide me in the shelter of his tabernacle and set me high upon a rock"* (v.5).

Friend, when you are armed with the Spirit and stand on God's Word, it doesn't matter what is swirling on the outside, the Lord will protect you in His tabernacle.

What a difference it makes when the Almighty arises within you: *"Then my head will be exalted above the enemies who surround me; at his tabernacle will I sacrifice with shouts of joy; I will sing and make music to the Lord"* (v.6).

GOD'S HOUSE IS THE ULTIMATE SHELTER - A DIVINE PLACE THAT CANNOT BE PIERCED BY SATAN'S ARROWS.

Think of David's situation. He was encircled by enemies, yet he could still praise God!

What a lesson for you and me. No matter how impossible the circumstances may seem, block them out and lift up your head. Begin to rejoice in the Lord. He is *"joy unspeakable and full of glory"* (1 Peter 1:8).

125

Give Him praise and thanksgiving – it's divine therapy!

Like A Bulldog

Why don't more people walk in the blessings of God? I believe it is because *they* give up before the *Son* comes up!

YOU HAVE TO BE TENACIOUS IN ORDER TO BE VICTORIOUS.

You have to be tenacious in order to be victorious. It's a principle that has been lost in our culture. In our "make-it-happen-fast" society, we want immediate results. For example, if the doctor prescribes a medication and it doesn't solve the problem in 24 hours we are on the phone complaining: "I don't understand. This stuff isn't working!"

I've learned a few lessons from, of all things, my little bulldog. If he decides he wants something, absolutely nothing is going to deter him. He's stubborn and extremely determined.

That's what the Lord expects from you and me:

- ■ He tells us to *"Hold on to instruction, do not let it go; guard it well, for it is your life"* (Proverbs 4:13).

126

- God says: *"Test everything. Hold on to the good"* (1 Thessalonians 5:21).
- He instructs us to *"hold on to our courage"* (Hebrews 3:6).
- Jesus says: *"I am coming soon. Hold on to what you have, so that no one will take your crown"* (Revelation 3:11).

The ultimate champions in the battle between life and death, heaven and hell, are those who reach out for the Lord, hang on and refuse to let go. The Bible says: *"They overcame him by the blood of the Lamb and by the word of their testimony; they did not love their lives so much as to shrink from death"* (Revelation 12:11).

It Pays!

Are you wiling to abandon *everything* to follow the Lord? Will you "lay it on the line" to stand with God's Son?

It's a risk worth taking, because your Father says that even if you lose, it will all be given back to you – not just in heaven, but in this life!

WILL YOU "LAY IT ON THE LINE" TO STAND WITH GOD'S SON?

Peter once said to Jesus, *"We have left everything to follow you!"* (Mark 10:28).

Here was the Lord's response: *"No one who has left home or brothers or sisters or mother or father or children or fields for me and the gospel will fail to receive a hundred times as much in this present age ...and in the age to come, eternal life"* (vv.29-30).

Serving Jesus Pays Great Dividends!

The next time someone infers, "It costs too much to follow Jesus," ask them to read this verse. Serving Jesus pays great dividends!

"Why Are You Doing This?"

Even the Apostle Paul, who endured incredible suffering because he proclaimed Christ, received a great reward.

At Lystra, a crippled man who was lame from birth was in the audience where he preached. The Bible records, *"He listened to Paul as he was speaking. Paul looked directly at him, saw that he had faith to be healed and called out, 'Stand up on your feet!' At that, the man jumped up and began to walk"* (Acts 14:9-10).

This caused a great uproar in this idol-worshiping city. Some of the locals even wanted to offer sacrifices to Paul and Barnabus. But Paul rushed into the crowd and declared, *"Men, why are you doing this? We too are only men, human like you. We are bringing you good news, telling you to turn from these worthless things to the living God, who made heaven and earth and sea and everything in them"* (v.15).

Also in the audience were some Jews from Antioch and Iconium who *"won the crowd over. They stoned Paul and dragged him outside the city, thinking he was dead"* (v.19).

Total Commitment

What was Paul's response? He stood up, dusted himself off and moved on to the town of Derbe, where they continued preaching the Good News and *"won a large number of disciples"* (v.21). He even returned to Lystra to tell the people, *"We must go through many hardships to enter the kingdom of God"* (v.22).

> **"WE ARE...STRUCK DOWN, BUT NOT DESTROYED."**
> - 2 CORINTHIANS 4:9

Through it all, Paul could say, *"We are hard pressed on every side, but not crushed; perplexed, but not in despair; persecuted, but not abandoned; struck down, but not destroyed"* (2 Corinthians 4:8-9).

Nothing – absolutely nothing – could tear Paul away from the love of the Father. He writes: *"For I am convinced that neither death nor life, neither angels nor demons, neither the present nor the future, nor any powers, neither height nor depth, nor anything else in all creation, will be able to separate us from the love of God that is in Christ Jesus our Lord"* (Romans 8:39).

What a shining example of total commitment!

Forever Changed

Why was Paul able to bear great persecution, yet rally again and again to preach the Gospel? It was because of his life-altering experience on the road to Damascus.

Saul (his former name) – who made murderous threats against the followers of Christ – was riding along on his horse when *"suddenly a light from heaven flashed around him. He fell to the ground and heard a voice say to him, 'Saul, Saul, why do you persecute me?'"* (Acts 9:3-4).

"SUDDENLY A LIGHT FROM HEAVEN FLASHED AROUND HIM."

- ACTS 9:3

"Who are you?" Saul asked.

"I am Jesus, whom you are persecuting," He replied. (v.5).

Saul was struck blind by the incident. At the Lord's direction, he was led by his friends to a house in Damascus where Anainas placed his hands on Saul and said, *"The Lord – Jesus, who appeared to you on the road as you were coming here – has sent me so that you may see again and be filled with the Holy Spirit"* (v.17).

Immediately the scales fell from Saul's eyes and he could see again. He rose up and was baptized.

From that moment Saul – who became the Apostle Paul – was forever changed. He was no longer groping in darkness. The sun had risen and he had a burning desire to tell the world about Jesus.

JUST ONE WORD FROM JESUS MAKES THE DIFFERENCE!

Neither the onslaughts of Satan or the physical attacks on Paul's body could slow him down. He was energized from above. As Jesus declared: *"The Spirit gives life; the flesh counts for nothing. The words I have spoken to you are spirit and they are life"* (John 6:63).

Just one word from Jesus makes the difference!

The Heat Was On!

Paul wasn't the first, nor the last, to be tested.

Do you recall what happened to the three Hebrew children who refused to bow to the golden image King Nebuchadnezzar had set up? Even though there was a decree that whoever fails to fall down and worship the image would be thrown into a blazing furnace, Shadrach, Meshach and Abednego adamantly refused.

Furious with rage, the king summoned the three to come before him and explain their disobedience. What was their answer? "Oh, Nebuchadnezzar," they replied, *"we do not need to defend ourselves before you in this matter. If we are thrown into the blazing furnace, the God we serve is able to save us from it, and he will rescue us from your hand, O king. But even if he does not, we want you to know, O king, that we will not serve your gods or worship the image of gold you have set up"* (Daniel 3:16-18).

After this heart-felt confession of their faith, the king *"ordered the furnace heated seven times hotter than usual"* (v.19). And the three were thrown into the flames.

The King was Amazed!

It's not much different today. When you make a uncompromising stand for Christ, the unbelievers who are not in tune with the Spirit are going to make it *hot!*

DON'T WORRY! THE LORD KNOWS WHERE YOU ARE AND WILL COME TO YOUR RESCUE.

Don't worry! The Lord knows where you are and will come to your rescue. That's what He did for Shadrach, Meshach and Abednego. When the king looked into the roaring flames, he was amazed and confused – and asked his advisers, *"Weren't there three men that we tied up and threw into the fire?"* (v.24).

They replied, "Certainly, O king."

He exclaimed, *"Lo, I see four men loose, walking in the midst of the fire, and they have no hurt; and the form of the fourth is like the Son of God"* (Daniel 3:25 KJV).

In the midst of the inferno, Jesus arrived! And the three walked out unscorched. Praise God, they didn't bow, didn't bend, and didn't burn!

Some people are like chameleons – adapting to their immediate surroundings, agreeing with everyone about anything, anytime, anywhere. They need to know that *"the cowardly, the unbelieving...the idolaters and all liars – their place will be in the fiery lake of burning sulfur. This is the second death"* (Revelation 21:8).

For them, it will be too late.

The Ransom

Today, before Christ returns for His church, you can be rescued and restored. No matter how far you may have fallen, or how dreadful the circumstances of your life, the Lord can cause the sun to shine once more.

If you think your situation is beyond redemption, start reading the Book of Job – the story of a man the Lord allowed Satan to test.

SOME PEOPLE ARE LIKE CHAMELEONS - ADAPTING TO THEIR IMMEDIATE SURROUNDINGS.

Listen to how Job was described: *"His flesh wastes away to nothing, and his bones, once hidden, now stick out. His soul draws near to the pit, and his life to the messengers of death"* (Job 33:21-22).

None of that mattered to Job. He had already made this declaration: *"Though he slay me, yet will I trust in him"* (Job 13:15 KJV).

Now, close to death, God sent an angel – a messenger – to him, saying, *"I have found a ransom for him"* (Job 33:24).

He Received Both a Double Portion and a Youthful Portion!

By faith, *"his flesh is renewed like a child's; it is restored as in the days of his youth. He prays to God and finds favor with him, he sees God's face and shouts for joy; he is restored by God to his righteous state"* (vv.25-26).

Job was about to be young again! Even more, the Lord caused him to prosper – *"and gave him twice as much as he had before"* (Job 42:10). God also added years to his life: *"After this, Job lived a hundred and forty years; he saw his children and their children to the fourth generation"* (v.16).

He received both a *double* portion and a *youthful* portion!

New Wings

Perhaps there are days you feel just like the elderly woman in the television commercial who says, "I've fallen and I can't get up!"

The help you need is not coming from a home security alarm system, you need to call out to God! Even if it seems you are trapped in a living hell, you don't have to accept it. As I told my congregation recently, "Just put a little 'o' on the end of hell and say *'Hello'* to your miracle!"

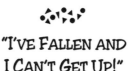

"I'VE FALLEN AND I CAN'T GET UP!"

Here's a verse to place on your refrigerator or on the dashboard of your car: *"Many are the afflictions of the righteous: but the Lord delivereth him out of them all"* (Psalm 34:19).

Memorize those words and repeat them again and again. You may be suffering, but the Lord is going to deliver you!

Remember, you can't stop what God has started, or destroy what He has promised.

Instead of complaining, start praising! Raise your voice and say: *"Bless the Lord, O my soul, and forget not all his benefits: Who forgiveth all thine iniquities; who healeth all thy diseases; Who redeemeth thy life from destruction; who crowneth thee with lovingkindness and*

135

tender mercies; Who satisfieth thy mouth with good things; so that thy youth is renewed like the eagle's" (Psalm 103:2-5 KJV).

Now you're ready to soar!

Healed and Strong!

What the Lord provided for the children of Israel, He will do for you! The Bible records: *He brought them forth also with silver and gold: and there was not one feeble person among their tribes"* (Psalms 105:37 KJV).

DOCTORS WEREN'T NEEDED IN THE WILDERNESS - THE SICK WERE HEALED AND THE WEAK BECAME STRONG.

Doctors weren't needed in the wilderness – the sick were healed and the weak became strong. God gave them such strength they were able to walk 'til the sun came up.

How do we know that? The Bible says, *"He guided them with the cloud by day and with light from the fire all night"* (Psalms 78:14).

The Lord hasn't changed. You are serving the God of Abraham, Moses and Elijah! He is:

- El Shaddai – God Almighty (Genesis 17:1).
- Jehovah Jireh – Our Provider (Genesis 22:14).
- Elohim – The Strong One (Jeremiah 32:27).

136

The prophet Isaiah asked: *"Do you not know? Have you not heard? The Lord is the everlasting God, the Creator of the ends of the earth. He will not grow tired or weary, and his understanding no one can fathom. He gives strength to the weary and increases the power of the weak. Even youths grow tired and weary, and young men stumble and fall; but those who hope in the Lord will renew their strength. They will soar on wings like eagles; they will run and not grow weary, they will walk and not be faint"* (Isaiah 40:28-31).

THE SAME GOD WHO PARTS THE WATERS AND GIVES SIGHT TO THE BLIND CAN ALSO INSTILL NEW STRENGTH – AND NEW LIFE THROUGH HIS SON, JESUS.

The same God who parts the waters and gives sight to the blind can also instill new strength – and new life through His Son, Jesus.

The Secret of Youth

In every chapter of this book we have seen God's principles for regaining our spirit of youth, yet when Jesus walked this earth He shared the one secret that makes it possible.

As the Lord was ministering in Judea, people started

bringing little children to Him so that He would touch and bless them. The disciples, however, began to push them away.

When Jesus saw what was happening He became indignant and said, *"Let the little children come to me, and do not hinder them, for the kingdom of God belongs to such as these. I tell you the truth, anyone who will not receive the kingdom of God like a little child will never enter it"* (Mark 10:14-15).

Next, He took the children in His arms, placed His hands on them and blessed their lives (v.16).

JESUS SAID, "YOU MUST BECOME YOUNG AGAIN IF YOU WANT TO ENTER MY KINGDOM."

The Lord wasn't saying "It's a good idea to regain your youth," or "I will help you add energy and zest to your life." He declared to the disciples and others who were listening something far greater. Jesus said, "You *must* become young again if you want to enter My Kingdom."

It is not an option. Salvation isn't the result of human logic or personal endeavor – it can only be received through childlike faith. And the Kingdom may only be entered by those who come to Christ without claim or merit.

A New Beginning

As adults, we rarely take things at face value. If we are presented with a concept or an idea, we ask: "When, where, who, what, and why?"

Children, however, believe what they hear. It you tell your son or daughter you're taking them to Disney World, they get excited and have faith in your promise.

That's exactly how you receive the greatest gift ever offered to man – the gift of salvation through the shed blood of Jesus.

HE WILL ROLL BACK THE CLOCK AND GIVE YOU A BRAND NEW BEGINNING.

When you become young in your faith, God will do something even more amazing. He will roll back the clock and give you a brand new beginning. Yes, you will be born again!

You may ask, "Is that truly possible?"

That's what a Pharisee named Nicodemus wanted to know. He came to Jesus at night and said, *"Rabbi, we know you are a teacher who has come from God. For no one could perform the miraculous signs you are doing if God were not with him"* (John 3:2).

Jesus ignored the flattery and got right to the point. He told the Jewish leader, *"I tell you the truth, no one can see the kingdom of God unless he is born again"* (v.3).

Nicodemus questioned, *"How can a man be born when he is old?...Surely he cannot enter a second time into his mother's womb to be born!"* (v.4).

The Lord explained that no one can enter the Kingdom of God unless he is born of water and the Spirit. Then He told Nicodemus these life-changing words: *"For God so loved the world, that he gave his only begotten Son, that whosoever believeth in him should not perish, but have everlasting life"* (v.16 KJV).

From Your Heart

If you have never asked Christ to come into your heart and forgive your sin, I would love to pray with you.

Right now – with childlike faith – say these words to the Lord:

God, I recognize that I have not lived my life for You up until now. I have been living for myself and that is wrong. I need and want You in my heart. I acknowledge the completed work of Your Son Jesus Christ in giving His life for me on the Cross at Calvary, and I long to receive the forgiveness you have made freely available to me through this sacrifice. Come into my life now, Lord. Take up residence in my heart and be my King, my Lord, and my Savior. From this day forward, I will no longer be controlled by sin, or

the desire to please myself, but I will follow You
all my days. I ask this in Jesus' precious and holy
name. Amen."

I rejoice with you that you have prayed these words
from your heart. You are a new creature in the sight of
God.

The first thing I recommend is that you tell someone
else about your new faith in Christ. Then spend time with
the Lord every day. It doesn't
have to be an extended period,
but develop the daily habit of
praying to Him and reading
His Word. Ask the Lord to
increase your faith and your
understanding of the Bible.

❖❖❖
I BELIEVE YOUR
LONG, DARK NIGHTS
ARE OVER.

Now seek fellowship with
other Christians by finding a local church where you can
worship God. Take the opportunity to follow Christ in
water baptism. Find a group of believers who will answer
your questions and support you.

It is the start of an exciting life!

You're Young Again!

Friend, I believe your long, dark nights are over. God
makes this promise: *"But unto you that fear my name*
shall the Sun of righteousness arise with healing in his

141

wings (Malachi 4:2 KJV).

Not only will the Lord arise, He is going to touch your heart, soul and mind, and make you like new. I love the final portion of that scripture: *"And you will go out and leap like calves released from the stall"* (v.2).

I can see it now! Tomorrow morning you are going to roll out of bed and start jumping for joy, shouting, "Praise God, I'm saved! I am healed and I'm on my way to heaven!"

You are young again!

FOR A COMPLETE LIST OF BOOKS, TAPES
AND OTHER MATERIALS, OR TO SCHEDULE
THE AUTHOR FOR CONFERENCES, SEMINARS AND
SPEAKING ENGAGEMENTS, CONTACT:

BISHOP ALAN H. MUSHEGAN
GOSPEL HARVESTER WORLD OUTREACH CENTER
1521 HURT ROAD
MARIETTA, GA 30008

PHONE: 770-435-1152
INTERNET: www.gospelharvester.com